Parkinson's Disease in Focus

IN FOCUS series

The *In Focus* series is a group of introductory texts to the pharmaceutical care of patients with chronic conditions.

Pharmacy can play a large part in the management of chronic conditions and titles in the *In Focus* series provide practical information on the pharmaceutical care, medication and management of patients.

Each title includes an introduction to the condition; signs, symptoms and diagnosis; prevention and management; monitoring and treatment (including alternative treatments); care of the patient and the future.

Aimed at practising pharmacists in hospital and community, these introductory books will also be helpful to pre-registration and undergraduate pharmacy students, and healthcare professionals with an interest/working in the field of the specific chronic disease.

Available titles in the series:
Asthma in Focus, *Anna Murphy*
Schizophrenia in Focus, *David Taylor*
Diabetes in Focus, 2nd edition, *Anjana Patel*
Osteoporosis in Focus, *Niall Ferguson*
Parkinson's Disease in Focus, *Charles Tugwell*
Stroke in Focus, *Derek Taylor*

Parkinson's Disease in Focus

Charles Tugwell

BPharm, MSc, ACPP, MRPharmS, MCLIP

Senior Directorate Pharmacist for Head and Neck Services, and
Clinical Pharmacist for Neurology and Neurosurgery
Barts and The London NHS Trust
London, UK

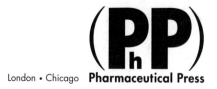

London • Chicago **Pharmaceutical Press**

Published by the Pharmaceutical Press
An imprint of RPS Publishing

1 Lambeth High Street, London SE1 7JN, UK
100 South Atkinson Road, Suite 200, Grayslake, IL 60030-7820, USA

© Pharmaceutical Press 2008

(**PP**) is a trade mark of RPS Publishing

RPS Publishing is the publishing organisation of the Royal
Pharmaceutical Society of Great Britain

First published 2008

Typeset by Type Study, Scarborough, North Yorkshire
Printed in Great Britain by TJ International, Padstow, Cornwall

ISBN 978 0 85369 696 4

A catalogue record for this book is available from the British Library

To Irene for providing inspiration and encouragement, and having unlimited patience during the writing of this book

Contents

The colour plate section is between pages 110 and 111.

Preface

Parkinson's Disease in Focus is written for healthcare practitioners who have a particular involvement with patients suffering from the condition. It is also intended as a textbook suitable for undergraduate and postgraduate students of pharmacy and medicine. The book is written in such a way that patients themselves, as well as their families and carers can also get much useful information from it and build upon their understanding of the disease, its management and the treatments available.

Parkinson's Disease in Focus opens with an introductory chapter followed by one on the condition, including its prevalence, aetiology, pathophysiology and its diagnosis. Signs and symptoms are described, paving the way for later chapters where management and treatment of the disease are discussed in some detail. Chapter 3 covers the pharmaco-therapy of Parkinson's disease, examining each of the key drug groups in turn as well as providing an outline for the approach to treatment. Non-drug therapies such as physiotherapy, speech and language therapy and occupational therapy play a major part in the overall management of Parkinson's disease. Chapter 4 provides an overview of these therapies and also gives details of complementary therapies to which a large number of patients attach high importance. It is appropriate therefore that this book includes information on complementary therapies, not only for patients but for healthcare professionals who often have little knowledge of these other forms of treatment. Surgical procedures for treating Parkinson's disease have been used for many years. In suitable patients, surgery provides a further approach when drug therapy is unsatisfactory and symptoms remain uncontrolled. Chapter 5 discusses the various surgical options and the use of deep brain stimulation. Too often, insufficient consideration is given to the non-motor symptoms suffered by patients with Parkinson's disease. Sometimes these may in fact be more troublesome and reduce quality of life more than the motor symptoms commonly associated with the disease. Chapter 6 reviews the range of potential symptoms that may occur as discussed in earlier chapters, and outlines the treatments that may be helpful. Much research into Parkinson's disease is underway and hopefully as understanding of the condition increases so will the development of new treatments. Avenues of research currently being explored are discussed in Chapter 7. In addition to new drugs affecting neuronal transmission, the chapter covers the potential for neuro-protective/neurorestorative agents, gene therapy, the use of stem cells and tissue transplantation. Chapter 8 looks at practical aspects of service provision and patient care. The recently published national guidelines on Parkinson's disease and the *National Service Framework for Long Term Conditions*, which mainly focuses on neurological illnesses, are summarised. The results of a project carried out in community pharmacies are discussed. This project was designed to determine the potential contribution that pharmacists can make to the care of patients with Parkinson's disease. This is followed by some aspects of pharma-ceutical care that are particularly relevant to this group of patients. A case study is also included in this chapter and readers are recommended to read through this since it pulls together a number of key issues discussed in the book. Students of pharmacy or medicine should perhaps work out and propose appropriate 'answers' to the various parts of the case study before reading the explanations outlined in the pages that follow. This will provide valuable practice for examinations! A large number of organisations and websites exist to provide information and support to patients, their carers, and those working in healthcare. Details of a number of these are provided in Chapter 9. Finally, the book contains four appendices. The first consists of extracts from James Parkinson's original essay describing the condition and his recom-mended treatment. These extracts are very readable and will be of great interest to those interested in the historical aspects of the disease; the details given of the recommended treatment are intriguing! The second and third appendices summarise the key interactions that can occur with the drugs used to treat Parkinson's disease and the adverse effects these drugs can cause. The fourth appendix provides useful information about driving and Parkinson's disease – helpful for patients and their health-care practitioners alike when discussing this issue.

Ultimately, it is hoped this book will help readers to improve the quality of care for patients suffering with Parkinson's disease by increas-ing knowledge and understanding of the clinical management of this condition.

Charles Tugwell
September 2007

Acknowledgements

I am grateful to the many sufferers of Parkinson's disease that I have had the privilege to meet over the years who have shared with me their feelings about the condition and given me an insight to their illness, in particular my colleague and friend Richard Charvet, who I knew long before the disease struck, for providing first-hand experience as he moved from a state of good health to one severely affected by the disease as it followed its inevitable course.

I thank fellow-pharmacist Kai-Loke Chan for reading through the manuscript and identifying areas that warranted further explanation or clarification, as well as spotting numerous typographical errors. I also thank Louise McIndoe, Christina De Bono, Tamsin Cousins, Penny Howes and Calum Ross at the Pharmaceutical Press for their tremendous help and guidance during the preparation of this book.

About the author

Charles Tugwell has worked at The Royal London Hospital, which is part of Barts and The London NHS Trust, for nearly 30 years. At the time of writing this book, he was Principal Pharmacist for Active Medicines Information Services in the trust, Clinical Pharmacist in Neurology/Neurosurgery and the Directorate Pharmacist for Clinical Neurosciences. In the spring of 2007 he took up the post of Senior Directorate Pharmacist for Head and Neck Services.

Charles developed a particular interest in neurological conditions and their treatment soon after starting work at The Royal London Hospital in 1978. His experience in this clinical area has been evolving ever since, working with both inpatients and outpatients. He has a special interest in the management of conditions such as Parkinson's disease, multiple sclerosis and epilepsy, and is a member of the Department of Health's Long-term Conditions NSF Stakeholder Group.

Focus points

Abbreviations

ADL	activities of daily living
AHP	allied health profession
AHPwSI	allied health professionals with special interest
AMPA	alpha-amino-3-hydroxy-5-methyl-4-isoxazole-propionic acid
CAT	computerised axial tomography
CBD	corticobasal degeneration
CNS	central nervous system
COMT	catechol-O-methyl transferase
CSM	Committee on Safety of Medicines
CT	computerised tomography
DATATOP	Deprenyl and Tocopherol Antioxidative Therapy of Parkinsonism (study)
DBS	deep brain stimulation
DLB	dementia with Lewy bodies
DNDF	dopaminergic neurons differentiation factors
DVLA	Driver and Vehicle Licensing Agency
ECT	electroconvulsive therapy
EPDA	European Parkinson's Disease Association
ESR	erythrocyte sedimentation rate
ESS	Epworth Sleepiness Scale
FDA	Food and Drug Administration
GABA	γ-aminobutyric acid
GAD	glutamic acid decarboxylase
GDNF	glial cell line-derived neurotrophic factor
GP	general practitioner
GPi	globus pallidus interna
GPwSI	GP with special interest
hRPE	human retinal pigment epithelial cells
HRT	hormone replacement therapy
5-HT	5-hydroxytryptamine
IVF	*in vitro* fertilisation
LSVT	Lee Silverman Voice Therapy

LTC CGWT   Long Term Conditions Care Group Workforce Team
MAO   monoamine oxidase
MAOI   monoamine oxidase inhibitor
MARS   Medicine Adherence Report Scale
MHRA   Medicines and Healthcare Products Regulatory Agency
MPTP   1-methyl-4-phenyl-1,2,3,6-tetrahydropyridine
MRI   magnetic resonance imaging
MRS   magnetic resonance spectroscopy
MSA   multiple system atrophy
MUR   medicines use review
NICE   National Institute for Health and Clinical Excellence
NI-IPL   non-immunosuppressive immunophilin ligand
NMDA N-methyl-D-aspartate
NO   nitric oxide
NSF   National Service Framework
NUDS   Northwestern University Disability Scale
NwSI   nurse with special interest
OPCA   olivopontocerebellar atrophy
PCT   primary care trust
PDQ 39   Parkinson's Disease Questionnaire 39
PDSS   Parkinson's Disease Sleep Scale
PEG   percutaneous endoscopic gastrostomy
PET   positron emission tomography
PhwSI   pharmacist with special interest
PNF   proprioceptive neuromuscular facilitation
PSP   progressive supranuclear palsy
PSS   personal social services
PVP   posteroventral pallidotomy
PwSI   practitioner with special interest
RBD   REM sleep behaviour disorder
REM   rapid eye movement
RLS   restless legs syndrome
rTMS   repetitive transcranial magnetic stimulation
SAMe S-adenosylmethionine
SDS   Shy–Drager syndrome
SF 36   Short Form 36
SIMS   Satisfaction with Information on Medicines
SND   striatonigral degeneration
SOD   superoxide dismutase
SPECT   single photon emission computed tomography
SSRI   selective serotonin reuptake inhibitor

STN	subthalamic nucleus
TCEP	transcranial electric polarisation
THC	delta-9-tetrahydrocannabinol
TMS	transcranial magnetic stimulation
UPDRS	Unified Parkinson's Disease Rating Scale
UPSIT	University of Pennsylvania Smell Identification Test
VIM	ventrointermediate nucleus

1

Introduction

People are living longer. Since 1930 the number of people living beyond 65 years of age has more than doubled, and it has been estimated that the number of people reaching the age of 90 will double in just 30 years. Parkinson's disease is a condition that more often affects the older members of our society. The prevalence in the 60–69 age group is 1 in 300 and this increases threefold in the 70–79 age group to 1 person in every 100 suffering with the disease. The prevalence in age groups above this is even higher. Clearly, since Parkinson's disease most commonly affects the elderly, the number of sufferers will rise substantially in the years to come. In turn, the need for clinical and social services to care for and support patients with Parkinson's disease will increase at a rapid rate, with major implications for the resources that are allocated to healthcare.

Current estimates put the total average cost of caring for a patient with Parkinson's disease in the UK at £6000 annually, two-fifths of which is direct costs to the NHS. As newer drugs and surgical procedures become available, these costs are likely to rise. Of course, it is not only in the treatment of Parkinson's disease that new therapies will be found. As medicine advances, so will the need for funding in order to provide the new technologies to patients. Many of these developments will be for conditions with a higher incidence in older age such as Alzheimer's disease as well as many non-neurological conditions, adding further to the financial burden as people live for longer.

Much research is under way in an attempt to improve upon the treatments that we have today to treat Parkinson's disease. Ways of delaying progression of the disease or even reversing it are being sought. Perhaps research will even reveal measures that can be taken to prevent Parkinson's disease developing in the first place. This book focuses mainly on the clinical aspects of treating patients with Parkinson's disease, but clearly healthcare economies will be an important factor influencing provision of services and patients' access to them in an NHS that is already struggling to match patient need against available resource.

About Parkinson's disease

Parkinson's disease is a progressive disorder of the central nervous system. It is one of the most common neurological conditions and occurs with more or less equal frequency in all countries around the world. As discussed previously, it has a much higher incidence in older people. However, so-called 'young-onset' (between 20 and 40 years of age) and 'juvenile-onset' (less than 20 years of age) Parkinson's disease can occur, though thankfully much less frequently.

To many people, the term Parkinson's disease is synonymous to having a tremor. As this book describes, Parkinson's disease is much, much more than suffering with a tremor, though this is indeed one feature of the disease that occurs in the majority of patients. Equally, there are many causes of tremor apart from Parkinson's disease. There are also a number of conditions that can have such a similar presentation to that of true Parkinson's disease that they are called parkinsonian syndromes. The focus of this book is on idiopathic Parkinson's disease, though these other conditions are discussed in terms of their significance during the process of diagnosis.

Many famous people suffer (or have suffered) from Parkinson's disease. Perhaps in more recent years, Pope John Paul II has received the most publicity. Others to have succumbed to the condition include the evangelist Billy Graham; the singers Johnny Cash and Ozzy Osbourne; the poet John Betjeman; and the actors Kenneth More, Michael Redgrave and Michael Fox. The boxer Muhammad Ali is also often cited as a sufferer, though it is more likely he has pugilistic Parkinson's syndrome rather than idiopathic Parkinson's disease.

About James Parkinson

James Parkinson was born in 1755 in Shorditch. His father, John, was an apothecary and the fact he conducted his practice from the family home probably accounted for James's intention from a very early age to follow in his father's footsteps. At the age of 16 years he became an apprentice to his father, and as part of his training attended the nearby London Hospital (now The Royal London Hospital). He subsequently undertook a surgical apprenticeship, which he completed in 1778. At this time his father's health was deteriorating and James became a partner in the family practice. Over the following years, in parallel with his medical practice, James Parkinson became very interested and active in politics, feeling strongly the need for a change in the country's system of government. He also developed a deep interest in geology, writing a number of articles and even a textbook on the subject entitled *Organic Remains of a Former World*. But it is his publications on medical matters that are more relevant here; especially the one entitled *An Essay on the Shaking Palsy* (see Plate 1). In this he described a disorder of the nervous system which, much later, some 60 years after his death, was to be named after him.

Readers interested in medical history will be intrigued by his account of the disease (see Appendix A, page 189). Those with more of an interest in the clinical aspects of the disease will find his original text to be remarkably descriptive, especially considering that it was based on observations of just six people suffering with the condition. Although his description provides insight to his detailed observations, the final chapter of the publication, which gives advice on treatment, would, in relation to today's therapeutic options, give cause for concern. He advocates withdrawing blood from a vein in the neck and repeatedly applying irritant poultices until a purulent discharge occurs. Parkinson believed the disease was caused by the spinal cord becoming either swollen or compressed. The drastic treatment used for localised swelling was obviously considered a rational approach for what we now know to be an incorrect explanation for the cause of the condition. It is probably better we remember James Parkinson for his detailed descriptions of the disease rather than his prediction of its pathology or his recommended treatment!

2

The condition

Prevalence and incidence

Figures suggest that Parkinson's disease is slightly more common in men than women (ratio 1.2:1). In the UK, the overall prevalence (total number of cases at any point in time) is around 1 person per 500 of population, which equates to 120 000 cases. The prevalence of Parkinson's disease in people in their 60s is 1 in 300, and this increases dramatically to 1 in 80 in people aged 80 years or more.

It is uncommon for the disease to occur in those aged less than 40 years; when it does it is known as 'young-onset Parkinson's disease'. It very rarely occurs in people aged less than 20 years, but when it does it is referred to as 'juvenile-onset Parkinson's disease'.

The incidence of a disease reflects the number of new cases occurring over a set period of time, and unlike prevalence it is not affected by survival rates. In the UK, the figure is around 18 per 100 000 of population per year, which means approximately 10 000 new cases of Parkinson's disease are diagnosed annually.

Main signs and symptoms

Parkinson's disease can cause a broad spectrum of symptoms and there is significant variation between patients in the way the disease manifests and the speed with which symptoms develop. However, three symptoms are clearly fundamental to Parkinson's disease and often develop as the early signs:

- hypokinesia and bradykinesia
- rigidity
- tremor.

Invariably, these initially present as unilateral symptoms. If a patient is demonstrating bilateral symptoms early on, it is much less likely that the correct diagnosis is Parkinson's disease.

Hypokinesia and bradykinesia

Reduction in movement (hypokinesia) and slowed movement (brady-kinesia) lead to a general 'slowing down', and physical tiredness may be the first indication that a patient has the early stages of Parkinson's disease. The symptoms of poverty of movement may be so vague initially and the onset so gradual that the person puts it down to just 'getting old'. A substantial degree of disablement resulting from impaired motor function may occur before the person realises something else may be responsible and seeks advice. When a patient presents with these symptoms, often there is not only slowness of movement but also a progressive reduction in the amplitude of motor activity with develop-ing fatigue.

Hypokinesia (together with rigidity – see below) also results in a reduction of facial expression. The bland expression that patients with Parkinson's disease often have does little to help good communication, as it leads to misperceptions by others who either do not realise the person has Parkinson's disease or do not understand the symptoms associated with it. Other noticeable effects resulting from hypokinesia include a reduction or loss of arm swing when walking, and difficulty experienced in attempting to carry out fine movements.

Rigidity

The rigidity, or muscular stiffness occurring with Parkinson's disease exacerbates the problems with movement resulting from hypokinesia and bradykinesia. All muscle groups can become affected. The patient themself is usually unable to distinguish the contribution rigidity plays to their movement problems. The increase in muscle resistance occurs when there is passive movement of, for example, a relaxed limb when someone else moves it. When examining a patient, rigidity becomes apparent when their wrist is being bent or their head turned to the side. The resistance to passive movement is constant throughout the range of movement, unlike spasticity where sudden relaxation can occur after movement has begun.

If the patient also suffers with tremor, the so-called cogwheeling effect can be seen. This jerky movement results from the tremor super-imposed on top of the rigidity.

Tremor

Tremor is another of the main symptoms associated with Parkinson's disease. However, contrary to popular belief, it is not universal and approximately one-quarter of patients do not have tremor. The involuntary rhythmical shaking normally occurs at rest and tends to reduce or stop when the affected part is used for some activity, for example if the hand is reached out to take hold of something. However, sometimes the patient also has an 'action tremor', similar to that seen in patients with essential tremor. The tremor of Parkinson's disease is quite coarse with a frequency usually between 4 and 6 Hz. Although the hands are often affected, some patients experience tremor of the jaw or foot. The tremor affecting the thumb and first finger produces the commonly called 'pill-rolling' effect.

In approximately three-quarters of patients, tremor is the first symptom to be observed. However, since non-parkinsonian tremor can occur, it is important to differentiate between parkinsonian tremor and essential tremor. This is usually straightforward since essential tremor occurs when the patient is asked to maintain a posture or perform an action, while parkinsonian tremor occurs at rest, although, as mentioned above, this is not always the case.

Although most patients present complaining of trembling in one hand, if the history is probed more deeply it often comes to light that this was not in fact the first symptom to occur. Slowness, some loss of dexterity and a degree of awkwardness in carrying out some physical activities has often preceded the onset of a trembling hand. But patients frequently tolerate these signs without complaining. However it is often the development of tremor which patients find hard to ignore and leads to them seeking advice.

Other signs and symptoms

Postural instability

Patients with Parkinson's disease develop a characteristic flexed posture resulting especially from flexion of the knees and hands. As the course of Parkinson's disease progresses, postural instability becomes a more troublesome feature. A steady posture is normally maintained by the nervous system making continuous reflex adjustments. Impairment of these mechanisms leads to a reduced ability to maintain balance, making the patient less steady when walking and particularly when turning. This substantially increases the risk of falls. It has been estimated that two-thirds of patients with Parkinson's disease have a fall each year. Typically a patient develops a stooped posture and this, together with a shuffling movement of the feet when walking, leads to a forward festinating (involuntary quickening) gait.

Posture can be assessed by sharply pulling on the patient's shoulders from behind. In Parkinson's disease with postural instability, the patient will be unable to compensate and fall backwards. With normal control of balance, a person will take a step backwards to maintain an upright posture.

Gait symptoms are a common feature of Parkinson's disease, but usually occur around five years after initial diagnosis. Occurrence in the early stages of the disease is unusual, however in the elderly the development of gait problems tends to occur sooner compared to younger patients.

Freezing

'Freezing' is the term used to describe the situation where a patient is either unable to initiate movement or suddenly stops the flow of movement. This is sometimes triggered by an external factor such as entering through a doorway or narrow space.

Dysphagia

Dysphagia (difficulty in swallowing) is a common problem in up to one-half of patients, especially those in the more advanced stages of Parkinson's disease. The dysphagia can arise from a reduction in tongue movement passing food or saliva to the back of the throat, or difficulty in initiating the swallow. Clearly this can affect the ability to eat and drink and make the taking of medication troublesome. The problems with eating and drinking can be substantial and may inhibit the patient's willingness to eat in the presence of other people because of the embarrassment of continuous coughing, spluttering and choking. Aspiration of food into the lungs predisposes patients to chest infections. In very severe cases, malnutrition may occur.

Speech problems

There are many ways in which speech may be adversely affected by Parkinson's disease. Decrease in muscle movement of the larynx can reduce the volume and articulation of speech making it difficult for others to understand what is being said. This is compounded by the tendency for phrases to be said in a rush, the patient being unable to control the speed of delivery. Sometimes, long silences occur as a patient has difficulty starting the beginning of a sentence or new phrase. The loss of facial expression which also occurs in Parkinson's disease does little to aid the process of successful communication. The development of speech problems tends to occur at an earlier stage of the disease in older patients.

Depression

The significance of depression as a feature of Parkinson's disease is often underestimated. Nearly one-half of Parkinson's disease patients suffer with depression, and quality-of-life assessments have shown this symptom to be a major factor in reducing quality of life. Specific treatment for depression may not only improve mental wellbeing, but subsequently improve other symptoms that may have worsened with the development of depression such as sleep problems, fatigue, bradykinesia and tremor.

Hallucinations

Visual hallucinations are not an uncommon feature of Parkinson's disease, especially in older patients and those who have had the condition for a long time. Patients typically state that they can see images of people, animals or insects nearby. They may describe seeing other people in the room with them (sometimes 'little people'), and frequently they seem to disappear if the patient stares at them.

It is rare for the hallucinations experienced to be auditory, and the images normally remain silent. Perhaps surprisingly, patients with Parkinson's disease who have hallucinations do not usually find them particularly frightening or menacing. In fact some patients claim they feel companionship with the person or animal that is the subject of the hallucination. However, a small minority of patients do become very distressed and terrified with the hallucinations they experience, at the time believing the images to be real.

Unfortunately, some of the drugs used in the treatment of Parkinson's disease can themselves precipitate hallucinations as an adverse effect, the anticholinergic drugs and direct-acting dopamine agonists being the main offenders. If a patient starts to have hallucinations for the first time soon after starting new therapy, consideration should be given to this being the possible cause and drug treatment modified if necessary. It is also possible for other illnesses such as severe infection to cause hallucinations in susceptible people.

Dementia

Serious cognitive impairment occurs in about one-fifth of patients with advanced Parkinson's disease. Aspects of mental function such as reduced short-term memory, confusion, adverse effects on judgement and reasoning, and visual hallucinations are key features of dementia. It is important to bear in mind that dopaminergic drug therapy may exacerbate (or cause) these symptoms. In some cases, the development of dementia may result in the patient being admitted to hospital or care home. Such a move to new surroundings can, understandably, make symptoms even worse.

Handwriting

Micrographia, writing that is very small sometimes to the point of being unreadable, is often an early symptom of Parkinson's disease (see Figure 2.1). The writing becomes smaller and smaller the longer the patient writes. Although a patient's handwriting is rarely restored to normal, it is usually significantly improved by drug therapy for Parkinson's disease.

Sense of smell

Although a reduced sense of smell (anosmia) occurs in a high proportion of patients with Parkinson's disease, it is rare for them to notice the decrease or to refer to it when a history is being given. The diagnostic value of testing for anosmia is discussed on page 22.

Bladder problems

Nocturia (frequent urination at night) is often the first indication that Parkinson's disease is affecting the bladder. The symptom is usually mild and occurs in later stages of Parkinson's disease. Detrusor hyper-reflexia produces a sense of urgency and urinary frequency. Some patients notice that the problems are more common during the 'off' periods of Parkinson's disease. Since patients usually take less medication at night, more 'off' time occurs, which adds to the problems of bladder frequency at night. This in turn contributes to sleep problems. Anticholinergic

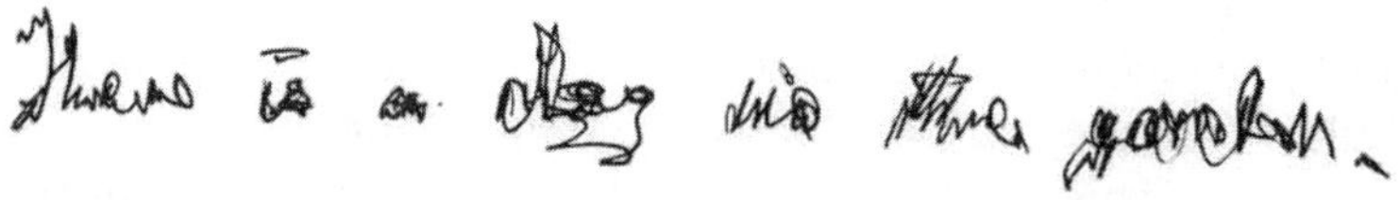

Sample of handwriting from a patient suffering with essential tremor prior to treatment of the condition

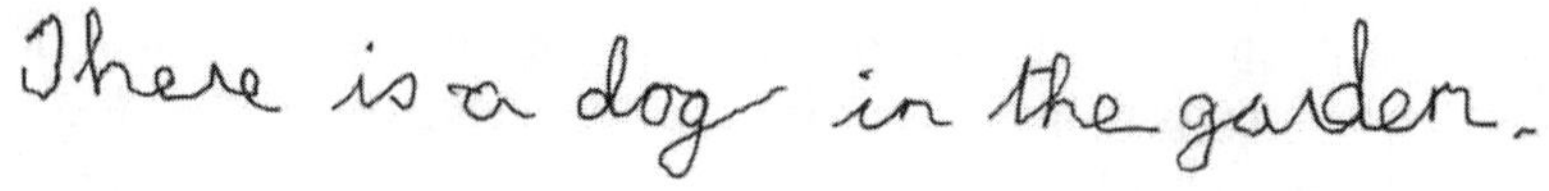

Sample of handwriting from the same patient writing the identical sentence following commencement of therapy with a beta-blocker for their essential tremor

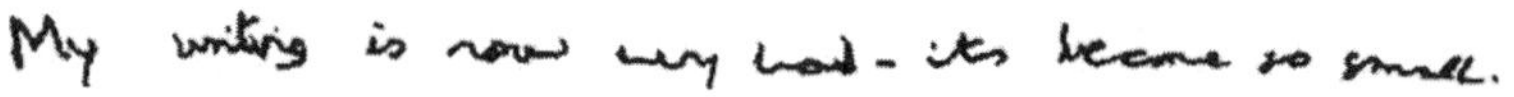

Sample of handwriting from a patient with Parkinson's disease

Figure 2.1   Essential tremor and Parkinson's disease can each produce substantial changes in a patient's handwriting, the characteristics of which are demonstrated above. Micrographia can be one of the early symptoms of Parkinson's disease and may be a useful observation in the diagnosis of the condition. Some improvement in writing may be seen after starting anti-Parkinson's drug therapy, though it rarely returns to normal. The use of rubber grips for pens can sometimes help.

drugs, which are less commonly used these days to treat Parkinson's disease, can produce the opposite effect, resulting in urinary retention.

Constipation

The main gastrointestinal symptom associated with Parkinson's disease is constipation, which affects a large proportion of patients. This is the result of reduced stool transit in the colon, but severity may be made worse by inadequate intake of liquid and food caused by swallowing difficulties (see previously). Constipation may cause abdominal distension, colicky pain and substantial discomfort. Pelvic floor muscle dystonia may affect the rectum and anus, which, instead of relaxing when trying to pass a stool, go into spasm. In this case, laxatives will not be helpful.

Sleep problems

Nearly all patients with Parkinson's disease report various disturbances with sleep. In the majority of cases, problems are the result of limb movements, myoclonic jerks or leg cramps. Being unable to turn over in bed during the 'off' period, as well as the tremor associated with Parkinson's disease can also interfere with sleep.

Sometimes more specific causes can be identified such as restless legs syndrome (RLS) or rapid eye movement (REM) sleep behaviour disorder (RBD), where motor activity occurs in parallel with dreaming.

Insomnia is often a symptom of depression and if this is the cause, antidepressant treatment will often be beneficial.

Other causes such as nightmares or vivid dreams can be associated with drug therapy used to treat Parkinson's disease.

Sexual problems

The physical aspects of Parkinson's disease such as bradykinesia and tremor can directly interfere with sexual function. Additionally, symptoms of depression may affect sexual function and decrease interest in sexual activity.

Aetiology

The cause of Parkinson's disease is not yet known, although as described in the following section, the area of the brain affected and some of the defective neuronal pathways have been established. Although research has so far been unable to identify the specific cause, a number of factors have been linked to the development of the disease. Some of these at least are likely to play a part either individually or in combination. It is conceivable that there is a variety of causes resulting in different types of idiopathic Parkinson's disease which have yet to be differentiated. Environmental and genetic factors have been widely studied and have been proposed as the precipitating cause of Parkinson's disease.

Environmental factors

For many years, the idea that exposure to environmental toxins such as certain pesticides may cause Parkinson's disease has received much attention. Indeed, some studies have shown there to be a significantly increased risk (albeit small) of Parkinson's disease in people with a higher exposure to pesticides, such as farmers. Some studies have also shown a higher incidence in people who drink water from wells.

Although itself unrelated chemically to any pesticides, MPTP (1-methyl-4-phenyl-1,2,3,6-tetrahydropyridine) has clearly been shown to cause symptoms of Parkinson's disease. This came to light in America when a chemistry graduate produced MPTP while attempting to create an analogue of pethidine as a 'designer drug' for selling to drug abusers. His entrepreneurial venture had disastrous consequences when the agent caused rapidly developing and severe symptoms of Parkinson's disease. Neuronal loss in the substantia nigra was shown at post mortem in those exposed to MPTP, which fits our understanding of the pathophysiology of the disease. MPTP has subsequently been used to good effect by pharmacologists in the laboratory. By inducing symptoms of Parkinson's disease with MPTP, a laboratory model can be created for researching new drugs to treat the disease. Similarities between the chemical structure of a metabolite of MPTP and that of the pesticide paraquat understandably led to concerns about the use of this agent (see Figure 2.2). However, evidence confirming any link between the toxic effects of paraquat and the development of Parkinson's disease is lacking.

Certain vitamins have been the subject of suspicion for an association with Parkinson's disease, especially an excess of vitamin E. However the evidence for this is so far poor. In contrast, it has been suggested that vitamin C decreases the risk of Parkinson's disease.

One of the most deeply researched environmental factors for Parkinson's disease is infection, both viral and bacterial. However, there is still no evidence from post mortems and serological tests that implicates bacterial or viral infection as a cause. That such efforts have been made to identify such a cause for the neurodegenerative process is understandable since an epidemic of encephalitis in the early 1900s was closely followed by a large outbreak of post-encephalitic parkinsonism.

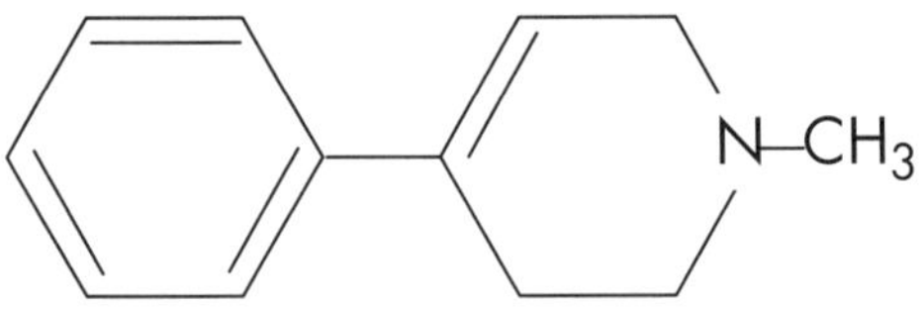

MPTP
(1-methyl-4-phenyl-1,2,3,6-tetrahydropyridine)

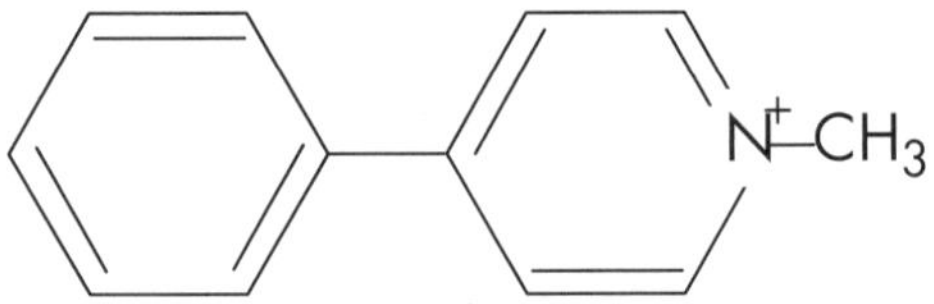

MPP^+
(MPTP metabolite)

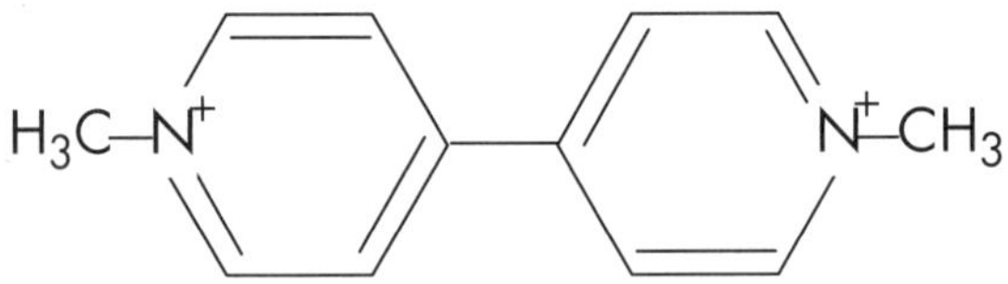

Paraquat

Figure 2.2 Chemical structures for MPTP (1-methyl-4-phenyl-1,2,3,6-tetrahydropyridine), MPP^+ (a metabolite of MPTP) and paraquat.

Genetic factors

In recent years, geneticists have accumulated increasing evidence of genetic defects associated with the development of Parkinson's disease. However, such monogenetic links have been found in very few families, and in the majority of cases Parkinson's disease is not thought to be directly inherited. Nevertheless, it has been estimated that having a parent with Parkinson's disease increases the lifetime risk of developing Parkinson's disease from 2% to 6%.

A number of genes have been identified as being implicated in Parkinson's disease, including those listed in Box 2.1. Most patients have no genetic cause for their Parkinson's disease. It is currently believed that only 5% of all cases of Parkinson's disease have a genetic cause.

> **Box 2.1** Genes identified for Parkinson's disease
>
> - alpha-nuclein (*PARK1*)
> - parkin (*PARK2*)
> - ubiquitin carboxy terminal hydrolase-L1 (*UCHL1*)
> - DJ-1 (*PARK7*)
> - *NR4A2*

A number of families around the world who have a very high occurrence of Parkinson's disease within-family have been found to have a gene defect. In these families the risk of a family member developing Parkinson's disease is increased by up to 50%. Mutation of the alpha-synuclein gene was the first to be linked to a dominantly inherited Parkinson's disease in a large Italian family. The fact that Lewy bodies found in the nerve cells of patients with Parkinson's disease have a high concentration of alpha-synuclein adds weight to the connection. The parkin gene has been associated with a juvenile-onset form of Parkinson's disease in some Japanese families.

The volume of information on malfunctioning genes connected to the occurrence of Parkinson's disease is rapidly increasing. In the years ahead this could lead to strenuous efforts to find forms of gene therapy that will rectify the defects in genes that may be responsible for Parkinson's disease. Even if Parkinson's disease is not directly inherited in the majority of patients, some form of genetic susceptibility may play a part and predispose to other (e.g. environmental) factors.

Pathophysiology

The basal ganglia

For many years, it has been known that the basal ganglia play a major role in regulating and controlling movement. Although many more parts of the jigsaw have been put in place, modern-day diagrams of the pathways involved with movement are still simplistic and far from complete. It is now accepted that the straightforward model used for many years to describe what goes wrong in Parkinson's disease and to explain the mode of action of anticholinergic drugs and levodopa is no longer applicable or helpful. This model (Figure 2.3) is based on a push–pull mechanism between acetylcholine and dopamine. When in balance, normal control of movement was possible; when out of balance due to decreased dopamine, symptoms of Parkinson's disease resulted.

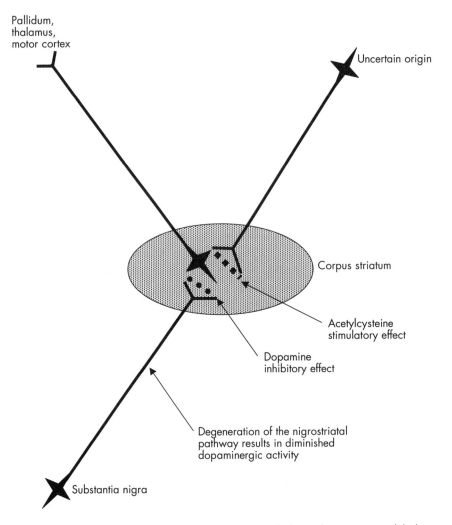

Figure 2.3 Early-day model describing the upset balance between acetylcholine and dopamine occurring in Parkinson's disease.

Despite the inadequacy of this explanation the starting premise is correct, i.e. that symptoms of Parkinson's disease result from degeneration of the dopaminergic pathway from the substantia nigra to the corpus striatum.

The following outline of the functional anatomy of the basal ganglia and the pathophysiology of Parkinson's disease is still inadequate, but is several steps closer than the model referred to above. Voluntary movement is controlled by the basal ganglia, which are a group of subcortical nuclei consisting of the:

- striatum (caudate and putamen)
- globus pallidus (externa and interna)
- substantia nigra (pars compacter and reticularis)
- subthalamic nucleus.

Pathways from these nuclei form loops between the motor cortex and the motor thalamus. No connections are made directly to descending pathways of the spinal cord. The loop system is made up of both excitatory and inhibitory pathways, the excitatory pathway passing via the subthalamic nucleus. The balance between the excitatory and inhibitory loops is modulated by the dopaminergic pathway from the substantia nigra. Activity of this pathway has been likened to that of a car accelerator, while activity via the subthalamic nucleus loop acts like a brake (see Plate 2).

The main neurotransmitters within these loops are glutamate and γ-aminobutyric acid (GABA). Glutamate is an excitatory neurotransmitter, while GABA is an inhibitory neurotransmitter. Plate 2 shows a complex interaction of excitatory and inhibitory neuronal pathways which, when operating normally, result in normal control of movement.

It is degeneration of the dopaminergic nigrostriatal pathway that occurs in Parkinson's disease resulting in an upset of this balance. This reduced activity, due to depleted dopamine, results in overactivity of the gabaminergic pathway running from the striatum to the globus pallidus (the striatopallidal pathway). As a consequence, excessive inhibition occurs on the pathway from the globus pallidus externa to the subthalamic nucleus. Since this too is a gabaminergic pathway, reduced inhibition occurs of the glutaminergic pathway running from the subthalamic nucleus to the globus pallidus interna. This reduced inhibition results in overactivity of the globus pallidus interna and increased firing of the gabaminergic neurons running from the globus pallidus interna to the thalamus. The excessive inhibition of the thalamus subsequently reduces stimulation of the motor cortex. Plate 3 illustrates this outcome, which stems from underactivity of the dopaminergic pathway between the substantia nigra and the striatum due to the degeneration that occurs in Parkinson's disease.

Lewy bodies

Lewy bodies, named after a German pathologist, are intracytoplasmic eosinophilic inclusions that are found in damaged neurons. Their presence within the pigmented brainstem nuclei is a feature of Parkinson's disease, although their role in the pathophysiology is still undetermined. It is unclear whether they are a result of the disease, or in some way involved in the cause of the pathology resulting in Parkinson's disease. It has been suggested they may be the result of a defective response to oxidative neuronal injury. Lewy bodies are found at post mortem in patients who have shown no signs of Parkinson's disease while alive. However, since symptoms of the disease do not manifest until substantial degeneration of the nigrostriatal pathway has occurred and dopamine levels in the striatum have fallen to around 20% of normal, it is conceivable that asymptomatic individuals who have Lewy bodies would have developed the disease had they lived longer. The prevalence of Lewy bodies in people with no signs of Parkinson's disease increases steadily with age, which corresponds to the age-related prevalence of the disease. Lewy bodies are found in patients with other neurodegenerative diseases including Alzheimer's disease, progressive supranuclear palsy (PSP) and multiple system atrophy (MSA). In dementia, the distribution of Lewy bodies is more widespread in the brain and they are found throughout the cerebral cortex. Although in Parkinson's disease Lewy bodies are predominantly present in the brainstem, their presence in peripheral autonomic nuclei may be associated with some of the autonomic features of the disease.

Oxidative stress

There is a growing body of evidence that oxidative stress plays some part in the pathogenesis of Parkinson's disease. Increased levels of iron are found in the substantia nigra and it is known that iron acts as a catalyst for oxidative reactions, which result in the production of free radicals. It is possible that neuronal damage is caused by an increase in oxidative stress resulting from an excess of free radicals. Free radicals are highly reactive since they contain one or more unpaired electrons. They oxidise other compounds by extracting electrons from them, often causing damage to the substances affected. Enzymes, other cellular proteins, deoxyribonucleic acid (DNA), and unsaturated fatty acids can all be damaged in this way. Examples of free radicals include: nitric oxide (NO); superoxide anion (O_2^-); hydroxyl radical (HO$^\bullet$); peroxynitrite (ONOO$^-$). The body produces other compounds such as superoxide dismutase (SOD) and glutathione peroxidase to 'scavenge' and 'neutralise' free radicals. Vitamin E, ascorbate and various other compounds can also destroy free radicals; hence the rationale behind some people trying vitamin E or vitamin C as a treatment for Parkinson's disease, though evidence for their clinical efficacy is lacking. Similarly iron-chelating agents seem to be ineffective. Further evidence that oxidative stress may be involved in Parkinson's disease is the increase in levels in the substantia nigra of chemicals indicative of lipid membrane damage and of 8-hydroxydeoxyguanosine, a product of DNA damage. The fact that the mitochondria of patients with Parkinson's disease have a substantially reduced activity of respiratory chain complex I, which would increase the opportunity for oxidative stress, adds further weight to the idea that oxidative stress and free radicals play a part in the pathophysiology of Parkinson's disease, albeit a poorly understood one.

Diagnosis and investigations

To correctly determine a diagnosis of Parkinson's disease, especially in the early stages, can present quite a challenge. As discussed earlier in this chapter, the trembling hand may be the symptom that triggers the patients to seek advice, but getting the patient to reflect on their wellbeing in recent months and years will sometimes identify other symptoms that they have previously disregarded or ignored. Such symptoms may include non-specific tiredness and general loss of energy, decreased dexterity (e.g. when dressing or using a computer keyboard accurately), taking longer to perform physical tasks, and increasing difficulty in writing. All of these can be early signs of the development of Parkinson's disease. Sometimes a patient may cite an activity or hobby which in recent times has become more difficult to pursue, such as swimming, dancing or running. Symptoms associated with early Parkinson's disease may be the cause for this. Occasionally, a patient will refer to other diagnoses that have been made in the past (incorrectly), such as rheumatic disease for what has been diagnosed as a frozen shoulder. Often, treatment for conditions such as this will have been prescribed.

Other symptoms that come to light when a patient is encouraged to think back may include what they describe as 'general aches and pains', 'getting old', increased sweating and feelings of 'shaking inside'. They may recall a single episode of what may be a relevant symptom that occurred some time back, such as a 'nervous breakdown' or a sleeping disorder. Looking back, a number of patients find that in the two or three years prior to the development of symptoms more specific to Parkinson's disease, they have become excessively emotional. All these things help to build up a picture that can be valuable in assessing the likelihood of accurately concluding a diagnosis of Parkinson's disease.

Unlike the diagnosis of many diseases, to conclude a patient has Parkinson's disease is not normally the result of assessing specific diagnostic tests. More often the diagnosis is determined from clinical observations, the presenting signs and symptoms, and to some extent the history as outlined on the previous page. Nevertheless, it can be difficult to distinguish idiopathic Parkinson's disease from certain other neurological conditions. It has been estimated that around 10% of patients are misdiagnosed even by neurologists and clinicians specialising in care of the elderly who are experienced in diagnosing and treating Parkinson's disease; this proportion of patients does not have the accepted pathological criteria for the condition. Approximately 5% of patients who *do* have pathology of Parkinson's disease (i.e. postmortem-proven Parkinson's disease) have not been diagnosed with the condition. These are patients with Lewy bodies and evidence of degeneration of dopaminergic neurons at post mortem. It is a widely held view that around one-half of patients referred to a movement disorder clinic with a provisional diagnosis of Parkinson's disease do not in fact have the condition. A number of studies have shown that misdiagnosis is often made in patients with essential tremor, vascular parkinsonism or other parkinsonian syndromes.[1] Studies of material from brain banks in the UK and Canada have shown an incorrect diagnosis was made in about 25% of patients. Other work suggests that of patients in the community who are taking anti-parkinsonian drugs, only three-quarters have a diagnosis of parkinsonism, and approximately one-half have clinically probable Parkinson's disease. Since the correct diagnosis of Parkinson's disease is important for both prognostic and therapeutic reasons, the identification of any secondary cause of parkinsonian symptoms such as side-effects of certain drugs or cerebrovascular disease, both of which can produce symptoms similar to those of Parkinson's disease, is essential. Differential diagnosis is therefore an important requirement before commencing specific therapy for Parkinson's disease. The recently published national guidelines for the diagnosis and management of Parkinson's disease in primary and secondary care recommend that patients with suspected Parkinson's disease should be referred, untreated, to a specialist with experience in the differential diagnosis of the condition.[2]

Differential diagnosis

Essential tremor is very common, with a prevalence ten times that of Parkinson's disease. Despite this, many patients with essential tremor are wrongly given the diagnosis of Parkinson's disease. The characteristics of the two conditions are different. Tremor associated with Parkinson's disease mainly occurs at rest and diminishes or stops during an action. In contrast, essential tremor occurs when performing an action. There are various other differences, which often makes it straightforward for clinicians with expertise in neurology to distinguish between essential tremor and Parkinson's disease.

Drug-induced parkinsonism can be produced by a number of medications. Unlike Parkinson's disease, both sides of the body are usually affected equally, and the progression of symptoms is much more rapid. Stopping the drug responsible leads to resolution in the majority of cases, but this may take a number of weeks, even months. The older phenothiazine neuroleptics were a common cause, but even the newer 'atypical' neuroleptics can precipitate parkinsonism, though the risk is much less. Focus on causes of Parkinsonism (2.1) lists drugs that have the potential to cause drug-induced parkinsonism.

FOCUS ON CAUSES OF PARKINSONISM 2.1

Drugs that may produce parkinsonism
• Cinnarizine
• Flunarizine
• Pethidine
• Sodium valproate
• Amiodarone
• Lithium
• Methyldopa
• Metoclopramide
• Phenothiazines
• Calcium-channel blockers
• Selective serotonin reuptake inhibitors (SSRIs)

Parkinson's plus syndromes are a group of conditions that have a presentation very similar to Parkinson's disease, often making it impossible for experienced neurologists to differentiate them from Parkinson's disease (see Focus on causes of Parkinsonism (2.2)). Sometimes it may be some years after an initial diagnosis of Parkinson's disease has been made that the appearance of other symptoms alerts to the possibility of a Parkinson's plus syndrome. These syndromes tend to respond less well to anti-Parkinson's drug therapy, which may sometimes be a trigger to review the initial diagnosis.

FOCUS ON CAUSES OF PARKINSONISM 2.2

Parkinson's plus syndromes and other causes of parkinsonian symptoms

Parkinson's plus syndromes

- Multiple system atrophy (MSA)
  - Shy–Drager syndrome (SDS)
  - striatonigral degeneration (SND)
  - olivopontocerebellar atrophy (OPCA)
- Progressive supranuclear palsy (PSP)
- Corticobasal degeneration (CBD)
- Dementia with Lewy Bodies (DLB)

Other causes of parkinsonian symptoms

- Essential tremor
- Drug-induced parkinsonism (see Focus on causes of Parkinsonism (2.1))
- Alzheimer's disease
- Wilson's disease
- Multiple cerebral infarct state
- Trauma (pugilistic encephalopathy)
- Toxins (carbon monoxide, manganese, copper, MPTP)
- Hyperthyroidism (tremor)

Olfactory function (smell testing)

Hyposmia (reduced sense of smell) is thought to be present in a high proportion of patients with Parkinson's disease,[3] and the idea that testing a patient's sense of smell could be helpful in confirming a diagnosis is being pursued. Whether smell-testing techniques will be helpful in distinguishing between Parkinson's disease and parkinsonism syndromes remains to be seen, though there is some evidence that it may be possible to distinguish Parkinson's disease from vascular parkinsonism.[4] There is evidence that hyposmia is associated with true Parkinson's disease and dementia with Lewy bodies, whereas patients with other parkinsonian conditions have a normal sense of smell. The diagnostic value of this feature of the disease is under-utilised, and smell testing should be carried out more frequently since it may help differentiate Parkinson's disease not only from vascular parkinsonism, but also from PSP and CBD. Two different tests can be used to assess olfactory function – UPSIT (University of Pennsylvania Smell Identification Test) and the 'sniffin sticks' test. Oregano (one of the smells in the UPSIT test) seems particularly valuable in determining anosmia in patients with Parkinson's disease. However, it is probably not essential to use these formalised testing schemes in order to gain a useful indication of whether a patient has hyposmia. More-routinely available items on a ward such as an orange will often suffice.

Investigations

As yet, there is no simple test that enables confirmation of an accurate diagnosis of Parkinson's disease. However, a number of techniques and forms of brain imaging may be used, mainly in specialist centres to assist in diagnosis. In practice, apomorphine and levodopa challenge tests help little in differential diagnosis between Parkinson's disease and various Parkinson's plus syndromes, and are rarely performed. There is evidence that anal sphincter electromyography is able to differentiate Parkinson's disease from similar conditions and is sometimes used to confirm a diagnosis of MSA.

Imaging techniques have been developed over the years and have contributed much to the current knowledge of the pathophysiology of Parkinson's disease. As research tools they have been valuable and on occasions provide useful techniques for helping with the task of diagnosis.

Computerised tomography (CT) scans appear normal in Parkinson's disease, but may show areas of atrophy in MSA. The main value of performing a CT scan is in excluding other conditions such as hydrocephalus, or small strokes as evidenced by areas of tissue damage.

Magnetic resonance imaging (MRI) scans have a higher resolution and can be valuable in assisting the diagnosis of PSP as well as MSA. Images are produced by applying high-strength magnetic fields which excite hydrogen atoms in water molecules.

Positron emission tomography (PET) scans are able to give an idea of cell functioning, whereas CT and MRI scans show structural changes that may be present in the brain. PET scans enable uptake of dopamine by the dopaminergic neurons of the nigrostriatal pathway to be measured (see Plate 4). A positron-emitting radioactive marker is administered to the patient, such as ^{18}F-6-fluorodopa (^{18}F-dopa). When taken up by presynaptic dopaminergic neurons in the caudate and putamen (corpus striatum) it is metabolised to ^{18}F-dopamine. Emission of positrons by the isotope enables tissue concentrations to be measured. At present, PET scans are mainly used in research and at specialist centres since special scanning equipment is needed which is not so readily available in hospitals (compared to SPECT scans – see page 24). PET scans are also expensive.

Single photon emission computed tomography (SPECT) scans (also known as Dat scans) are cheaper to carry out and are more readily available in hospitals, and therefore in practical terms are sometimes used and can provide helpful results. These scans do not use tracers specific for measuring dopamine storage; ^{99m}technetium and ^{123}iodine are the isotopes more commonly used. Labelled derivatives of cocaine, ^{123}I-β-CIT and ^{123}I-FP-CIT, are most frequently used with SPECT. These target presynaptic dopamine reuptake sites. The gamma-ray-emitting isotope enables visualisation of uptake in the caudate and putamen, which is reduced in Parkinson's disease and certain other conditions. This form of scanning is not able to confirm a diagnosis of Parkinson's disease, MSA or PSP, but may be helpful in distinguishing other conditions such as vascular parkinsonism. Normally a SPECT scan will show good uptake of the tracer in the putamen and caudate, whereas in Parkinson's disease, uptake will be decreased. Therefore it can be useful in confirming a patient does *not* have Parkinson's disease. Normal scans are produced in certain types of parkinsonism, for example that resulting from an adverse effect of drug therapy such as calcium channel blockers, neuroleptic drugs and sodium valproate, since the area affected is the striatum rather than the nigra.

Patients with Huntington's disease, hydrocephalus or supratentorial tumours presenting with parkinsonism will usually have a normal SPECT scan as will those who have parkinsonian symptoms as a result of the toxic effects of carbon monoxide or manganese. Essential tremor and tremors that do not involve the presynaptic dopaminergic system result in normal uptake of tracer, and a scan can therefore be useful if it is not possible to distinguish tremors that may be due to Parkinson's disease from those caused by other conditions. However, it is possible that some cases of true Parkinson's disease can produce a normal SPECT scan which may therefore be misleading.

UK clinical criteria for diagnosis

Generally speaking, the diagnosis of Parkinson's disease is based on clinical findings. It is therefore important that there are agreed criteria on which such a diagnosis can be made with a fair degree of certainty that it is correct. Clearly, the ultimate level of proof which can only be obtained at post mortem is of little practical use either for the patient or those seeking to treat them. The United Kingdom Parkinson's Disease Society Brain Bank has advocated a set of criteria that should be applied when diagnosing the condition (see Box 2.2).[5] Accuracy in diagnosis has

Box 2.2 United Kingdom Parkinson's Disease Society Brain Bank criteria for the diagnosis of Parkinson's disease[5]

Step 1: Diagnosis of a parkinsonian syndrome
Bradykinesia and at least one of the following:
- muscular rigidity
- rest tremor (4–6 Hz)
- postural instability unrelated to primary visual, cerebellar, vestibular or proprioceptive dysfunction

Step 2: Exclusion criteria for Parkinson's disease
A history of:
- repeated strokes with stepwise progression
- repeated head injury
- antipsychotic or dopamine-depleting drugs
- definite encephalitis and/or oculogyric crises on no drug treatment
- more than one affected relative
- sustained remission
- negative response to large doses of levodopa (if malabsorption excluded)
- strictly unilateral features after three years
- other neurological features: supranuclear gaze palsy, cerebellar signs, early severe autonomic involvement, Babinski sign, early severe dementia with disturbances of language, memory or praxis
- exposure to known neurotoxin
- presence of cerebral tumour or communicating hydrocephalus on neuroimaging

Step 3: Supportive criteria for Parkinson's disease
Three or more required for diagnosis of definite Parkinson's disease:
- unilateral onset
- rest tremor present
- progressive disorder
- persistent asymmetry affecting the side of onset most
- excellent response to levodopa
- severe levodopa-induced chorea
- levodopa response for over five years
- clinical course of over 10 years

implications not only for appropriate management, but also for the prognosis, which is better for patients with Parkinson's disease compared to those with MSA or PSP.

Measuring the severity of symptoms

Several rating scales have been developed in order to assess the severity of Parkinson's disease and the degree of impact the condition has on carrying out everyday tasks. These scales are useful not only for measuring changes in a patient's condition, but also for objectively measuring the benefits of drug therapy in clinical trials. The fact that patients' symptoms can fluctuate widely needs to be taken into account when applying these scales in practice. The assessment made while a patient is in an 'off' phase will be very different from that made when the patient is 'on'.

Hoehn and Yahr clinical rating scale

This scale is mainly used to indicate the stage of a patient's disease based on the severity of the symptoms they are experiencing. Table 2.1 provides a summary of the scale. It is one of the more simple scales in use, but is not particularly sensitive in showing changes in a patient's functional ability.

Table 2.1   Hoehn and Yahr clinical rating scale

Stage	Severity
1.0	Tremor or rigidity on one side of the body only (with or without bradykinesia)
1.5	Tremor or rigidity on one side of the body and axially (with or without bradykinesia)
2.0	Moderate tremor or rigidity on both sides of the body with bradykinesia but no impairment of balance
2.5	Moderate tremor or rigidity on both sides of the body with bradykinesia, but recovery on retropulsion (pull) test
3.0	Significant tremor or rigidity on both sides of the body with bradykinesia and some postural instability (patient still physically independent)
4.0	Severe disability, but still able to stand and walk without assistance
5.0	Bedridden or wheelchair bound unless assisted (patient unable to function independently)

Unified Parkinson's Disease Rating Scale (UPDRS)

This more extensive scale assesses over 40 aspects of the disease (see Table 2.2). Not only are aspects of motor function assessed and the ability to perform everyday tasks, but other symptoms such as dysphagia

Table 2.2 Unified Parkinson's Disease Rating Scale (UPDRS)

Part	Severity
I	Mentation (4 items)
II	Activities of daily living (13 items)
III	Motor function (14 items)
IV	Complications of treatment (11 items)

and mental wellbeing are also covered. The UPDRS provides a framework for scoring the spectrum of symptoms that can be associated with Parkinson's disease and is commonly used in clinical trials to measure the effectiveness of various drug treatments.

Schwab and England Scale

This scale primarily focuses on the level of disability and assesses a patient's degree of independence. The measure is expressed in terms of a percentage from 100%, which reflects complete independence and the

Table 2.3 Schwab and England rating scale

Percentage	Description
100	Fully functioning; tasks performed with no difficulty; patient completely independent
90	Some tasks take longer due to a degree of slowness and impairment; patient still completely independent
80	Difficulty in performing some tasks; significant slowness; patient still completely independent
70	Substantial slowness in performing tasks; some tasks quite difficult; patient no longer completely independent
60	Very slow in performing tasks; some tasks now impossible; much effort required; patient now partly dependent on other people
50	Difficulty in performing many tasks; needs assistance with bathing etc.; patient now dependent on other people
40	Unable to carry out many tasks without help; patient now very dependent on other people
30	Can only carry out very few tasks without help; patient now highly dependent on other people
20	Unable to carry out any tasks alone; severely disabled; patient now nearly completely dependent on other people
10	Unable to carry out any tasks; completely disabled; patient now totally dependent on other people

ability of the patient to function normally, to 10%, where the patient is so badly affected that their degree of disability means that they are completely dependent upon other people. The Schwab and England scale is summarised in Table 2.3.

Activities of Daily Living Scale (ADL)

The Activities of Daily Living (ADL) Scale focuses on the everyday tasks and symptoms that may affect a patient's ability to perform them. Box 2.3 summarises the key areas covered by this assessment scale.

Box 2.3 Activities of Daily Living (ADL)

This scale measures the impact of Parkinson's disease on 14 categories:
- speech
- salivation
- swallowing
- handwriting
- cutting food and handling utensils
- dressing
- hygiene
- turning in bed and adjusting bedclothes
- falling
- freezing when walking
- walking
- left-sided tremor
- right-sided tremor
- sensory symptoms

Parkinson's Disease Sleep Scale (PDSS)

Sleep problems occur in a very high percentage of patients with Parkinson's disease. A scale has been developed to specifically measure the extent and impact that sleep problems cause.[6] A visual analogue scale is used to assess 15 symptoms associated with disturbed sleep in Parkinson's disease (see Box 2.4). The patient marks along the scale from 0 (severe symptoms and always experienced) to 10 (symptoms not experienced) for each of the 15 items included in the assessment. A scale such as this may be of particular value in assessing the effectiveness of treatments aimed at treating specific symptoms that disturb sleep such as restless leg syndrome.

Box 2.4 The Parkinson's Disease Sleep Scale (PDSS)

For each of the 15 items below, the patient indicates their response on a 10 cm line marked from 0 to 10, where 0 represents the worst score and 10 an excellent or never response.

Overall quality of night's sleep
1. How does the patient rate the quality of their sleep at night?

Sleep onset and maintenance
2. How easily does the patient fall asleep?
3. Does the patient stay asleep or keep waking up?

Nocturnal restlessness
4. Does the patient have restlessness of the arms or legs disrupting sleep?
5. Does the patient fidget in bed?

Nocturnal psychosis
6. Does the patient have distressing dreams?
7. Does the patient suffer with hallucinations at night?

Nocturia
8. Does the patient need to get up to pass urine?
9. Is the patient incontinent of urine because 'off' periods at night stop them getting up to pass urine?

Nocturnal motor symptoms
10. Does the patient wake up at night because of tingling or numbness in arms or legs?
11. Does the patient have painful muscle cramps in the arms or legs?
12. Does the patient wake early in the morning with painful posturing of the arms or legs?
13. Does the patient experience tremor when waking in the morning?

Sleep refreshment
14. Does the patient feel tired and sleepy after waking in the morning?

Daytime dozing
15. Does the patient unexpectedly fall asleep during the day?

Other scales

A number of other scales have been developed over the years including the Webster scale and the Northwestern University Disability Scale (NUDS), both of which consist of a number of items that are assessed to give a measure of impaired functionality and disability. Various quality-of-life scales have been used, which require the patient to rate a range of indicators reflecting their view on how they are affected due to impairment and disability. Examples of these include the Parkinson's Disease Questionnaire (PDQ 39), which is made up of 39 items; the Short Form 36 (SF 36), which is made up of 36 items; and the EuroQol (EQ 5).

References

1. Tolosa E, Wenning G, Poewe W. The diagnosis of Parkinson's disease. *Lancet Neurol* 2006; 5: 75–86.
2. National Institute for Health and Clinical Excellence. *Parkinson's Disease: diagnosis and management in primary and secondary care.* Clinical guideline 35. London: National Institute for Health and Clinical Excellence, 2006. www.nice.org.uk/CG035 (accessed 5 June 2007).
3. Double KL, Rowe DB, Hayes M, *et al.* Identifying the pattern of olfactory deficits in Parkinson's disease using the brief smell identification test. *Arch Neurol* 2003; 60: 545–549.
4. Katzenschlager R, Zijlmans J, Evans A, *et al.* Olfactory function distinguishes vascular parkinsonism from Parkinson's disease. *J Neurol Neurosurg Psychiatr* 2004; 75: 1749–1752.
5. Gibb WRG, Lees AJ. The relevance of the Lewy body to the pathogenesis of idiopathic Parkinson's disease. *J Neurol Neurosurg Psychiatr* 1988; 51: 745–752.
6. Chaudhuri KR, Pal S, DiMarco A, *et al.* The Parkinson's disease sleep scale: a new instrument for assessing sleep and nocturnal disability in Parkinson's disease. *J Neurol Neurosurg Psychiatr* 2002; 73: 629–635.

Further reading

Burch B, Sheerin F. Parkinson's disease. *Lancet* 2005; 365: 622–627.

Nutt JG, Wooten GF. Clinical practice. Diagnosis and initial management of Parkinson's disease. *N Engl J Med* 2005; 353: 1021–1027.

Suchowersky O, Reich S, Perlmutter J, *et al.* Practice parameter: diagnosis and prognosis of new onset Parkinson disease (an evidence-based review): report of the Quality Standards Subcommittee of the American Academy of Neurology. *Neurology* 2006; 66: 968–975.

3

Pharmacotherapy

Approach to treatment

There is currently no form of pharmacotherapy available that has been shown to delay the progression of Parkinson's disease. However, there exists a range of drugs that can treat the symptoms of the condition and consequently improve the patient's quality of life. Managing drug therapy in patients with Parkinson's disease can be complex. Although good control is often achieved in the early stages of the disease, as it progresses the drugs usually need careful tailoring with respect to choice of agents and combinations used, and dosage adjustments. These decisions are influenced by the degree of success and benefit achieved in an individual, and the development of adverse effects which can be a very significant factor.

In the very early stages of Parkinson's disease, when functional disability is minimal, the use of anti-Parkinson's drugs is often unnecessary and in fact the potential side-effects may be more of a problem than the condition itself. However, once symptoms are troublesome, the decision to commence pharmacotherapy has to be reconsidered. Once symptoms warrant treatment, this is usually initiated with levodopa combined with a peripheral dopa decarboxylase inhibitor (benserazide or carbidopa), or a dopamine agonist. Levodopa therapy is certainly the most effective, but invariably leads to motor complications further down the line. Dopamine agonists are not quite so effective, but cause less motor complications, though a range of other adverse effects can cause problems. Although there is no clear-cut evidence that dictates the approach to treatment, many consider levodopa should be used as initial pharmacotherapy in all patients with severe symptoms and in all elderly patients. A non-ergot dopamine agonist should be used for the initial treatment of younger patients with less-disabling symptoms. A third form of therapy which may be suitable as an initial treatment in patients who have relatively mild symptoms is with monoamine oxidase type B (MAO-B) inhibitors. These drugs can delay the need for using levodopa and may be adequate in the early stages of Parkinson's disease for improving motor symptoms.

Other drugs used much less frequently as treatments for the early stages of Parkinson's disease include amantadine and anticholinergics. These should not be regarded as first-line forms of therapy, though anticholinergics and beta-blockers may very occasionally be suitable in patients with early-stage disease when tremor is the main feature. The various approaches to managing the early stages of Parkinson's disease are being assessed in the large UK PD MED trial currently under way (for more information see www.pdmed.bham.ac.uk). This will hopefully provide useful information comparing the use of levodopa, dopamine agonists and MAO-B inhibitors in early disease, not only from a clinical and quality-of-life perspective, but also in health economics terms.

As the disease progresses, tailoring therapy often becomes more of a challenge. Not only does the increased severity of the symptoms need addressing, but the management of motor complications caused by levodopa becomes an important aspect of a patient's pharmacotherapy. Dyskinesia and the wearing-off effects of levodopa are attributed to the pulsatile nature of dopamine receptor stimulation resulting from medication. Controlled-release preparations of levodopa may reduce motor fluctuations in some patients, though decreased absorption of the drug may in fact increase the time a patient is in the 'off' phase. Sometimes, satisfactory control is gained by combining immediate-release and controlled-release dosage forms.

Dopamine agonists, MAO-B inhibitors and catechol-O-methyl transferase (COMT) inhibitors are used in combination with levodopa therapy in the later stages of Parkinson's disease. This form of adjunctive therapy often regains control of symptoms and may allow a reduction in levodopa dosage if the drug is precipitating motor complications. A non-ergot dopamine agonist such as pramipexole or ropinirole should be used in preference to the older ergot-derived compounds which are more likely to cause serious toxic effects. Amantadine can be used to reduce dyskinesia in later Parkinson's disease.

In patients with extremely severe motor complications, apomorphine may be effective in reducing 'off' time and dyskinesia associated with later disease. This drug has to be administered either as an intermittent injection or a continuous subcutaneous infusion. Serious adverse effects can occur and it is only initiated by specialist units where appropriate levels of ongoing monitoring can be provided.

As with therapy during the early stages of Parkinson's disease, the results of formal studies do not provide evidence for a definitive

An algorithm outlining a possible approach to the drug therapy of Parkinson's disease

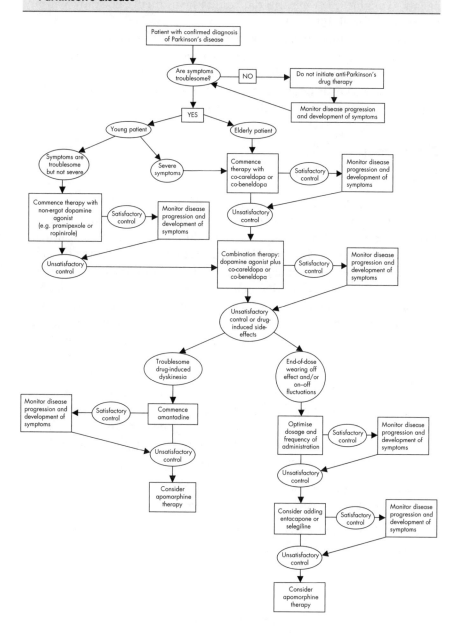

approach or a clear-cut drug of first choice in later Parkinson's disease. The UK PD MED trial may provide the necessary evidence enabling comparisons to be made between the various approaches to therapy and agents available. However, initial results from this large study will not be available until 2009/10.

The algorithm (Focus on pharmacotherapy (3.1)) provides a suggested overall approach to the pharmacotherapy of Parkinson's disease based on evidence currently available and practice in the UK. The various classes of drug and therapeutic options are discussed in more detail throughout the rest of this chapter.

Drug groups

Levodopa preparations

There can be few examples in medicine where the drug introduced nearly 40 years ago remains the mainstay of treatment today. But that indeed is the case with levodopa. Introduced around 1970 following initial work in the 1950s and 1960s, levodopa was to become the most effective treatment available to date. It was not until the late 1960s that Cotzias *et al.* used dosages that achieved the levels necessary to produce substantial improvement in motor impairment.[1] Although the beneficial effects on the symptoms of Parkinson's disease were dramatic, the high dosage needed invariably caused substantial nausea and vomiting. In the mid-1970s two agents were developed which inhibited the unwanted peripheral breakdown of levodopa. These agents enabled lower doses of levodopa to be used while maintaining its therapeutic effects in the central nervous system. The dosage reduction markedly decreased the problems with nausea and vomiting. Two preparations are available, each a combination of levodopa and one of the peripheral dopa decarboxylase inhibitors (see Figures 3.1–3.3):

- co-beneldopa   levodopa + benserazide (Madopar)
- co-careldopa   levodopa + carbidopa (Sinemet).

Since the 1980s, these two preparations have remained the most effective forms of drug treatment.

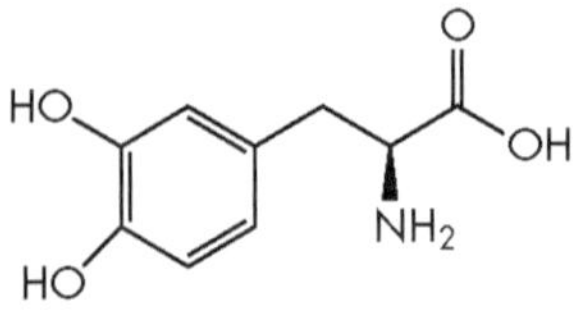

Figure 3.1   Levodopa.

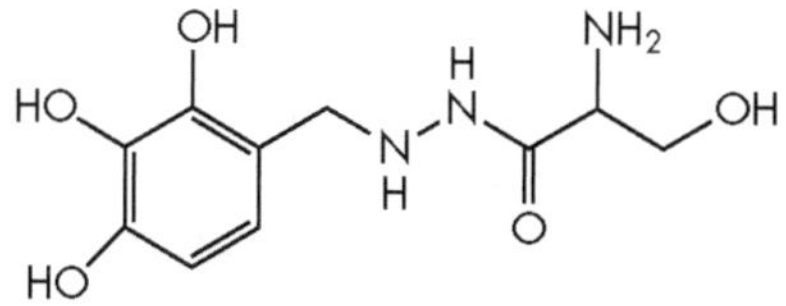

Figure 3.2   Benserazide.

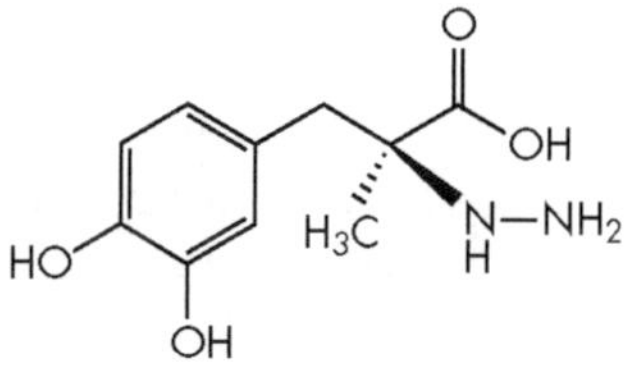

Figure 3.3   Carbidopa.

Levodopa is the precursor of the neurotransmitter dopamine which is deficient in certain parts of the brain responsible for the control of movement, particularly the nigrostriatal pathway. The enzyme dopa decarboxylase metabolises levodopa to dopamine both peripherally and centrally. The peripheral dopa decarboxylase inhibitor blocks peripheral conversion, but has no such effect centrally where the metabolism to dopamine is wanted in order to produce the desired pharmacological effect.

A large clinical study known as the ELLDOPA trial published in 2004, confirmed the widely held view that levodopa plus a peripheral dopa decarboxylase inhibitor is indeed a very effective treatment for Parkinson's disease.[2] Initial adverse effects are usually tolerated and in many cases are transient. The inevitable development of dyskinesias and motor fluctuations as treatment continues longer term is the main problem with what remains the most effective treatment available for Parkinson's disease. It is very rare for a patient who commences treatment with another drug for their Parkinson's disease not to eventually require the addition of levodopa.

Side-effects

Although nausea and vomiting caused by levodopa are much reduced with the combination preparations (levodopa + peripheral dopa decarboxylase inhibitor), these side-effects can still occur and are often troublesome for the first few weeks of treatment. Starting therapy at low dosage and reassuring the patient that these adverse effects are usually transient is often sufficient. In the more severe cases, domperidone (10 mg to 20 mg, three or four times daily) can be taken to reduce the severity of nausea/vomiting. Loss of appetite and postural hypotension are also common in the early weeks of treatment.

A variety of sleep disorders can occur, including insomnia, vivid dreams and nightmares. Taking the final dose of the day in early evening will reduce the likelihood of these problems. Visual hallucinations, confusion and delusions are more frequently encountered in the later stages of Parkinson's disease, either as a manifestation of the illness or because of the need to increase the dosage of levodopa.

Motor complications occur in a large proportion of patients who have taken levodopa for a number of years. Approximately half of patients on this form of therapy exhibit such effects after six years. These complications, which are normally irreversible, have led to the widely held view that levodopa should be held in reserve until symptoms of Parkinson's disease warrant commencing treatment with the drug, thus delaying the onset of these major motor side-effects. Such a policy is probably of more relevance to those patients who have Parkinson's disease diagnosed at an early age.

Dyskinesias (abnormal involuntary movements) often manifest as twisting of the limbs, trunk or face (athetoid movements), and jerky twitching of the limbs (choreiform movements). Two patterns of dys-kinesia can occur, the more common being peak-dose dyskinesia. This occurs when levodopa is producing maximum effect and is usually the first type of dyskinesia a patient develops. A decrease in dosage may sometimes reduce the problem in the short term, but in due course this fails to be helpful as adequate control of the symptoms of Parkinson's disease itself is lost. This situation is often worse for the patient than tolerating the dyskinesias. Similarly, subdividing the dosage further (taking less more frequently) does not help.

The other pattern of dyskinesia is known as biphasic. This occurs shortly after taking a dose (onset of effect) and when the effects are wearing off (end of dose). Plate 5 shows diagrammatically the pattern for both types of levodopa-induced dyskinesia. With biphasic dys-kinesia, the initial phase of dyskinesia is followed by an 'on' period without dyskinesia, but as the beneficial effects of the drug wear off a second phase of dyskinesia occurs. Taking a higher dose will prolong the time a patient remains above the threshold for dyskinesia to occur, but this is only successful as a short-term measure. Taking larger amounts of levodopa less frequently may decrease the length of time a patient is in the phase of dyskinesia. Sometimes patients only experience the onset phase, or only the end-of-dose phase. Many patients probably have a combination of peak-dose and biphasic dyskinesia. Dystonia is also common, the patient often adopting an unusual posture due to the severe and painful muscle contraction; this frequently occurs in the leg.

Further motor complications that arise from the long-term use of levodopa are fluctuations in response either from the 'end-of-dose' deterioration (wearing-off effect), or unpredictable on/off switching effect where patients switch between being mobile ('on') and immobile ('off') suddenly without warning.

There are various approaches to managing patients who are experiencing motor complications with levodopa therapy, but success is often the result of trial and error, and experience. Increasing the frequency of doses up to six or more times a day may be beneficial, supporting the belief that peak levels are responsible for the unwanted effects. Such a regimen may also decrease the incidence of end-of-dose deterioration. The use of modified-release preparations of co-careldopa and co-beneldopa may also be helpful. Alternatively, adjunctive therapy with a dopamine agonist or COMT inhibitor (see later) may be beneficial.

Modified-release preparations

In addition to immediate-release preparations of co-careldopa and co-beneldopa (see Focus on levodopa preparations (3.2 and 3.3)), each of

FOCUS ON LEVODOPA PREPARATIONS 3.2

Co-careldopa (Sinemet) tablets

Dosage (expressed as levodopa)

There are three alternative dosage regimens:

1
- initially 100 mg (with 25 mg of carbidopa as co-careldopa 25/100 (Sinemet-Plus)) three times daily
- increased by 50 mg to 100 mg (with 12.5–25 mg carbidopa as co-careldopa 12.5/50 (Sinemet 62.5) or co-careldopa 25/100 (Sinemet-Plus)) daily or on alternate days
- up to 800 mg (with 200 mg of carbidopa) daily in divided doses

or

2
- initially 50 mg to 100 mg (with 10–12.5 mg of carbidopa as co-careldopa 12.5/50 (Sinemet 62.5) or co-careldopa 10/100 (Sinemet 110)) three or four times daily

continued overleaf

Focus on levodopa preparations 3.2 (continued)
- increased by 50–100 mg daily or on alternate days
- up to 800 mg (with 80–100 mg of carbidopa) daily in divided doses

or

3
- initially 125 mg (with 12.5 mg of carbidopa as *half* a tablet of co-careldopa 25/250 (Sinemet 275) once or twice daily
- increased by 125 mg (with 12.5 mg of carbidopa) daily or on alternate days.

Notes
- *Transferring preparations*: if transferring from a different levodopa plus dopa decarboxylase inhibitor preparation, this should be stopped for at least 12 h beforehand. Treatment with co-careldopa should be started at a dose that provides the same amount of levodopa that the patient was previously taking.
- *Modified-release tablets:*
  - for initial treatment or to treat fluctuations in response, one MR tablet (co-careldopa 50/200 (Sinemet CR)) twice daily; both dose and interval adjusted according to response at intervals not less than 3 days
  - one MR tablet of co-careldopa 50/200 (Sinemet CR) twice daily can be substituted for a daily dose of 300–400 mg of levodopa as conventional co-careldopa tablets
  - if transferring from existing levodopa therapy, this is normally stopped 8 h beforehand.

Preparations

	Carbidopa	Levodopa
Tablets		
Co-careldopa 12.5/50 Sinemet 62.5	12.5 mg	50 mg
Co-careldopa 10/100 Sinemet 110	10 mg	100 mg
Co-careldopa 25/100 Sinemet-Plus	25 mg	100 mg
Co-careldopa 25/250 Sinemet 275	25 mg	250 mg
Modified-release tablets		
Co-careldopa 25/100 Half Sinemet CR	25 mg	100 mg
Co-careldopa 50/200 Sinemet CR	50 mg	200 mg

Note: Co-careldopa is also available in combination with the COMT inhibitor entacapone, see Focus on COMT inhibitors (3.15), page 73 for preparations available.

FOCUS ON LEVODOPA PREPARATIONS 3.3

Co-beneldopa (Madopar)

Dosage (expressed as levodopa)

- Initially 50 mg (100 mg in advanced disease) three or four times daily
- Increased by 100 mg once or twice weekly
- Usual maintenance dose 400–800 mg daily in divided doses

Notes

- *Elderly patients:*
  - in the elderly, the initial dose is usually 50 mg once or twice daily
  - increased by 50 mg every 3 or 4 days.
- *Transferring preparations:*
  - if transferring from a different levodopa preparation, this is normally stopped for up to 12 h beforehand
  - when transferring from another levodopa/dopa decarboxylase inhibitor preparation, the initial dose is usually 50 mg three or four times daily.
- *Modified-release capsules:*
  - in patients not previously receiving levodopa therapy, the initial dose is normally one capsule (100 mg of levodopa) three times daily
  - to treat fluctuations in response, one capsule (100 mg of levodopa) is substituted for every 100 mg of levodopa and given at the same frequency, increased every 2 or 3 days according to response; a 50% increase is typically needed above the previous levodopa dose, and titration may take up to 4 weeks.

Preparations

	Benserazide	Levodopa
Capsules		
Co-beneldopa 12.5/50 Madopar 62.5	12.5 mg	50 mg
Co-beneldopa 25/100 Madopar 125	25 mg	100 mg
Co-beneldopa 50/200 Madopar 250	50 mg	200 mg
Dispersible tablets		
Co-beneldopa 12.5/50 Madopar 62.5	12.5 mg	50 mg
Co-beneldopa 25/100 Madopar 125	25 mg	100 mg
Modified-release capsules		
Co-beneldopa 25/100 Madopar 125 CR	25 mg	100 mg

Note: the dispersible tablets may be swallowed whole or dispersed in water or orange squash, but not orange juice.

these combinations is available in a modified-release formulation. Co-beneldopa modified-release capsules (Madopar CR) form a gelatinous mass in the stomach which gradually releases its constituent drugs over 4–5 h, maintaining plasma levels for up to 8 h. The amount of drug absorbed is reduced by 30–40% compared to the immediate-release preparation. Co-careldopa has been formulated in a polymer-based matrix (Sinemet CR), which slowly erodes releasing levodopa and carbidopa. Absorption occurs over 4–6 h, and again bioavailability is reduced by approximately 30% compared to immediate-release co-careldopa. Unlike Madopar CR, the bioavailability of Sinemet CR is increased with food.

Intraduodenal administration

As discussed earlier in this chapter, treatment with levodopa will eventually lead to motor complications in the majority of patients including 'off' periods and substantial dyskinesias. It has been suggested that at least in part this is due to oral administration of levodopa producing widely fluctuating levels of dopamine in the patient, unlike the continuous supply of dopamine that occurs naturally in the healthy brain. Levodopa is primarily absorbed from the small intestine and it is likely that variable gastric emptying rates are the major cause of these fluctuating levels. Various studies have shown there to be a direct correlation between the variation in plasma levels and motor symptoms suffered by patients. One study has shown that large intra- and inter-patient variation occurs in mean plasma levodopa levels (between 0.45 and 7.07 µg/ml) and peak concentrations (between 0.95 and 13.75 µg/ml).[3] These fluctuations had a clear effect on the various clinical parameters assessed in the study.

After many years of research a gel of co-careldopa has been formulated specifically designed for continuous intraduodenal infusion via an external pump. Collaboration between the Departments of Neurology and Pharmacy at Uppsala University in Sweden has resulted in a stable suspension of micronised levodopa plus carbidopa in a methylcellulose gel (see Focus on levodopa preparations (3.4)).[4] Co-careldopa intestinal gel is now available in the UK as Duodopa (see Plate 6). Each 100 ml cassette of gel contains 2 g of levodopa plus 500 mg of carbidopa. A portable pump delivers the gel into the duodenum through a permanent tube via a PEG (percutaneous endoscopic gastrostomy). The dosage is individualised to produce optimal response for the patient. However, typically a morning dose of 5 ml to 10 ml (100 mg to 200 mg levodopa)

FOCUS ON LEVODOPA PREPARATIONS 3.4

Co-careldopa (Duodopa) intestinal gel for intraduodenal administration

---

Dosage (expressed as levodopa)
- Dosage is carefully adjusted to optimise the clinical benefit for each individual patient.
- A bolus dose, usually between 100 mg and 200 mg of levodopa (5–10 ml of gel) is given each morning.
- The maintenance dose is usually between 40 mg and 120 mg of levodopa (2–6 ml of gel) per hour.
- Extra bolus doses, usually between 10 mg and 40 mg of levodopa (0.5–2 ml of gel) can be administered.
- Normally, the maximum total daily dosage is less than 2 g of levodopa (one cassette).

Notes

- *Initial treatment:*
  - Duodopa should initially be given as monotherapy
  - a temporary nasoduodenal tube should be used initially to determine the likelihood of this form of treatment being successful.

Preparations

- Intestinal gel:
  - each 1 ml of intestinal gel (Duodopa) contains levodopa 20 mg and carbidopa 5 mg
  - the product is supplied in 100 ml cartridges.

Notes – storage:

- Duodopa cartidges need to be stored between 2°C and 8°C
- the shelf-life of Duodopa is limited to 15 weeks.

---

is administered, and a continuous maintenance dose between 2 ml and 6 ml (40 mg to 120 mg of levodopa) is infused. Extra bolus doses up to 2 ml (40 mg of levodopa) can be given during the day if required.

Administration in this way substantially reduces the variation in plasma levodopa concentrations compared with normal oral administration. A pharmacokinetic study in 16 patients showed plasma levodopa variance and coefficient of variation were significantly lower with Duodopa than with oral co-careldopa.[5] A non-blinded assessment from video recordings showed that patients on Duodopa spent more time in 'normal' motor state, less time in both 'off' and dyskinetic states compared with conventional therapy. Also, using a standard rating scale for assessing symptoms of Parkinson's disease (the UPDRS – Unified Parkinson's Disease Rating Scale) there was a statistically significant difference between the two administration methods.[5] In a more recent study, quality of life was shown to be significantly improved as assessed using two tools: the Parkinson's Disease Questionnaire 39 (PDQ 39) and the 15D Quality of Life Instrument.[6] Side-effects experienced from the intraduodenal gel were similar to those from oral therapy.

This form of treatment is only suitable for those patients who have advanced Parkinson's disease with severe motor fluctuations and in whom satisfactory control cannot be achieved with oral therapy or subcutaneous apomorphine (see later). It may offer a further option in those patients where other products are unsatisfactory and thoughts may be turning to a neurosurgical procedure because symptoms are so severe.

Dopamine agonists

Dopamine agonists directly stimulate postsynaptic dopamine receptors mimicking the pharmacological effects of the naturally occurring neuro-transmitter. A number of subtypes of dopamine receptor have been identified, though little is known about the various roles each plays within the central nervous system. The receptor types are divided into two families known as D_1 and D_2. The D_1 family consists of D_1 and D_5 receptors. The D_2 family consists of D_2, D_3 and D_4 receptors. Dopamine agonist drugs have significant affinity for receptors in the D_2 group, with apomorphine also having strong affinity for the D_1 group. The thera-peutic effects of these drugs results from their direct action on dopamine receptors in the pathways deficient of dopamine in the striatum as a result of Parkinson's disease.

Place in therapy

Adjunctive therapy

Oral dopamine agonists were introduced during the late 1970s as adjunctive therapy in patients receiving levodopa who had developed motor complications. A number of trials have shown that dopamine agonists can significantly reduce the 'off' time patients suffer. Adjunc-tive treatment may also allow a reduction in levodopa dosage and improvement in motor function. However, the extent of dyskinesia is often increased. A meta-analysis and review of trials carried out have not provided evidence of significant differences in clinical outcome terms between the drugs available in this group.

Monotherapy

Once the potential benefits of dopamine agonists as adjunctive therapy had been established, trials were carried out to determine their value as monotherapy. The results of these trials showed that dopamine agonists were as effective as monotherapy, certainly as initial therapy, until symptoms progressed making it necessary to add in levodopa. However, this is valuable since it can delay the need for commencing levodopa therapy which invariably leads to long-term problems associated with the drug such as 'on/off' fluctuations and dyskinesia. This is particularly important for younger patients who still have many years of life ahead of them.

For the purpose of this chapter, dopamine agonists have been divided into three groups:

1. ergot derivatives (bromocriptine, cabergoline, lisuride, pergolide)
2. non-ergot derivatives (pramipexole, ropinirole)
3. apomorphine.

Ergot derivatives

Four ergot derivatives are still used in the UK for treating Parkinson's disease: bromocriptine, cabergoline, lisuride and pergolide. They are used less frequently now that newer, non-ergot compounds are available which are potentially less toxic. All of the drugs listed above have been associated with the development of retroperitoneal fibrosis, pleural thickening and effusions, pericarditis and pericardial effusions. The Committee on Safety of Medicines (CSM) has advised continuous monitoring of patients on these drugs for signs and symptoms that may indicate the development of serious toxic effects.[7]

Bromocriptine

Bromocriptine (see Figure 3.4) has been regarded as the standard against which the effectiveness of adjunctive therapy with other dopamine agonists is measured. However, it is not commonly used these days in the treatment of Parkinson's disease, either as adjunctive therapy or monotherapy. Many patients find the side-effects troublesome and, as with all ergot-derivatives, potentially serious toxic effects can occur.

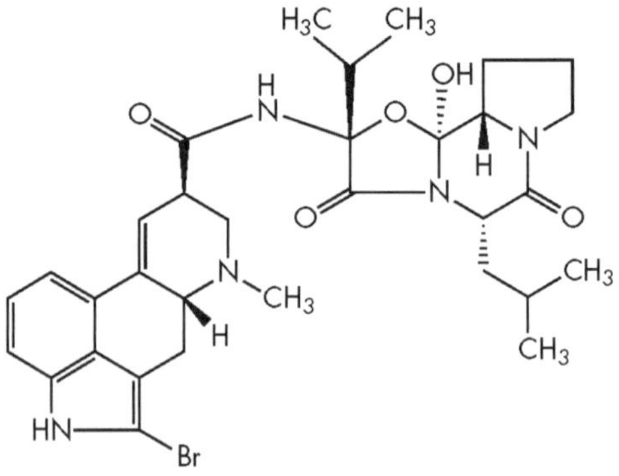

Figure 3.4 Bromocriptine.

Side-effects
See also under Ergot derivatives.

The most common side-effects that occur at the start of treatment are nausea, orthostatic hypotension and syncope. Since bromocriptine causes vasoconstriction, it can produce digital vasospasm in cold weather and leg cramps. Extra care is needed in patients with cardiovascular disease or Raynaud's syndrome. Headache, nasal congestion, dry mouth, constipation and diarrhoea can be troublesome. Also, psychosis, hallucinations, delusions and confusion are not infrequently encountered with the dosages used for treating Parkinson's disease.

Interactions
Erythromycin can increase the blood levels of bromocriptine, increasing the likelihood of dose-related side-effects. Alcohol and sympathomimetics such as phenylpropanolamine increase the risk of toxic effects.

The effects of bromocriptine may be antagonised by antipsychotics.

Pharmacokinetics
Bromocriptine is poorly absorbed (less than one-third of the dose taken). Bioavailability is further decreased by first-pass metabolism resulting in approximately 6% of the drug reaching the circulation. Up to 96% of the drug is protein bound. The main route of elimination is in the faeces. Bromocriptine is hydrolysed in the liver to lysergic acid and peptides, which pass back into the gastrointestinal tract via the bile.

See Focus on dopamine agonists (3.5).

FOCUS ON DOPAMINE AGONISTS 3.5

Bromocriptine

Dosage

- Week 1: 1 mg to 1.25 mg at bedtime
- Week 2: 2 mg to 2.5 mg at bedtime
- Week 3: 2.5 mg twice daily
- Week 4: 2.5 mg three times daily
- Thereafter:
  - increase by 2.5 mg every 3 to 14 days depending on response
  - usual maintenance dose is between 10 mg and 40 mg daily.

Notes

- *Food*: doses should be taken during a meal.
- *Stopping treatment*: when stopping dopamine agonist therapy, this should be done gradually.

Preparations

- Tablets of 1 mg bromocriptine (as mesilate) (Parlodel)
- Tablets of 2.5 mg bromocriptine (as mesilate) (Parlodel)
- Capsules of 5 mg bromocriptine (as mesilate) (Parlodel)
- Capsules of 10 mg bromocriptine (as mesilate) (Parlodel)

Note: 2.5 mg strength tablets are also available as a non-proprietary product.

Cabergoline

Cabergoline (see Figure 3.5) has similar effects to bromocriptine and as with this drug has D_2-agonist properties. It is used as adjunctive therapy in patients suffering from disabling 'on/off' motor fluctuations with levodopa. Patients who are unable to tolerate bromocriptine, may find that cabergoline causes them fewer problems. The reverse is also true.

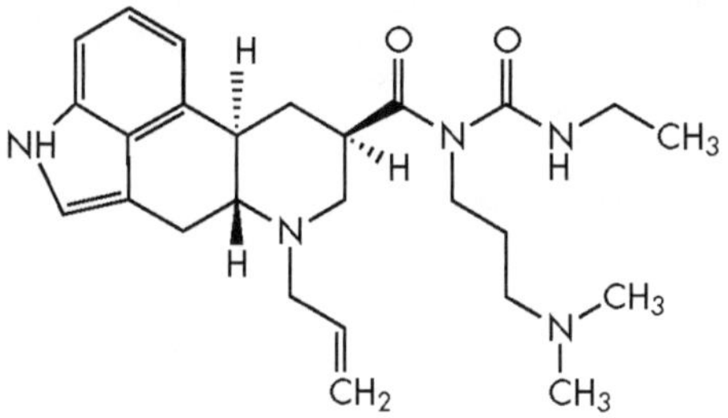

Figure 3.5   Cabergoline.

Cabergoline also has a longer duration of action which means the drug is taken less frequently.

Side-effects
See also under Ergot derivatives and Bromocriptine.

In addition to the side-effects cited for bromocriptine, cabergoline causes dyspepsia and gastritis in a significant number of patients. Adverse effects on the nervous system such as dyskinesia, hyperkinesia, hallucinations and confusion are the most commonly experienced.

Interactions
See Bromocriptine.

Pharmacokinetics
Cabergoline is rapidly absorbed from the gastrointestinal tract and is not significantly affected by the presence of food. It is almost entirely metabolised in the liver to what are believed to be inactive metabolites. These are primarily excreted in the faeces. The elimination half-life is particularly long – studies in healthy volunteers suggesting up to 68 h.

FOCUS ON DOPAMINE AGONISTS 3.6

Cabergoline

Dosage

- Initially 1 mg daily
- Increased by increments of 0.5–1 mg at 7- to 14-day intervals
- Usual maintenance dose is 2–6 mg daily

Notes

- *Food*: doses should be taken during a meal.
- *Stopping treatment*: when stopping dopamine agonist therapy, this should be done gradually.

Preparations

- Tablets of 1 mg cabergoline (Cabaser)
- Tablets of 2 mg cabergoline (Cabaser)
- Capsules of 4 mg cabergoline (Cabaser)

Note: 0.5 mg strength tablets are also available as Dostinex for the inhibition and suppression of physiological lactation and treatment of hyperprolactinaemic disorders.

It is estimated that steady-state levels are achieved after four weeks of dosing.

See Focus on dopamine agonists (3.6).

Lisuride

Lisuride (see Figure 3.6) can be used as monotherapy or as an adjunct to levodopa. However, the evidence supporting its use as monotherapy is poor and other agents are preferred. In the 1980s, studies were carried out using lisuride by subcutaneous and intravenous infusion for the treatment of motor fluctuations in Parkinson's disease. However, severe psychiatric symptoms occurred when the drug was administered by these routes.

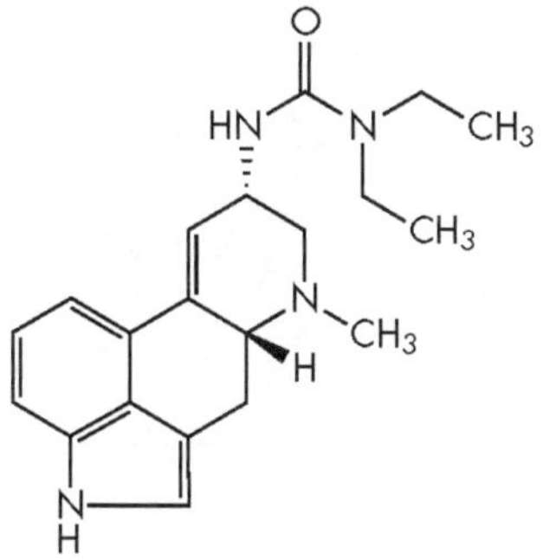

Figure 3.6   Lisuride.

Side-effects
See also under Ergot derivatives and Bromocriptine.

Lisuride can produce severe hypotension in some people. Nausea and vomiting, dizziness, headache and psychiatric effects are not un-common.

Interactions
See Bromocriptine.

Pharmacokinetics
Blood levels vary considerably between patients following oral adminis-tration of lisuride. Absorption appears to be rapid and the elimination half-life is approximately 2 h. Pharmacokinetic studies suggest that oral bioavailability varies according to the dose taken.

See Focus on dopamine agonists (3.7).

FOCUS ON DOPAMINE AGONISTS 3.7

Lisuride

Dosage

- Initially 200 μg at bedtime
- Increased at weekly intervals to:
  - 200 μg twice daily (at midday and bedtime)
  - then 200 μg three times daily (in the morning, at midday and bedtime)
- Thereafter, increase by 200 μg each week (adding firstly to the bedtime dose, then the midday dose and finally the morning dose)
- Maximum dose 5 mg daily in three divided doses

Notes

- *Food:* doses should be taken with food.
- *Stopping treatment:* when stopping dopamine agonist therapy, this should be done gradually.

Preparations

- Tablets of 200 μg lisuride maleate
- Available as a non-proprietary product

Pergolide

Like the other ergot derivatives, pergolide (see Figure 3.7) has D_1-agonist activity, but it also has effects on D_3 receptors. Pergolide is used both as monotherapy and as an adjunct to levodopa. Prior to the introduction of pramipexole and ropinirole, pergolide was often used as monotherapy in younger patients with Parkinson's disease.

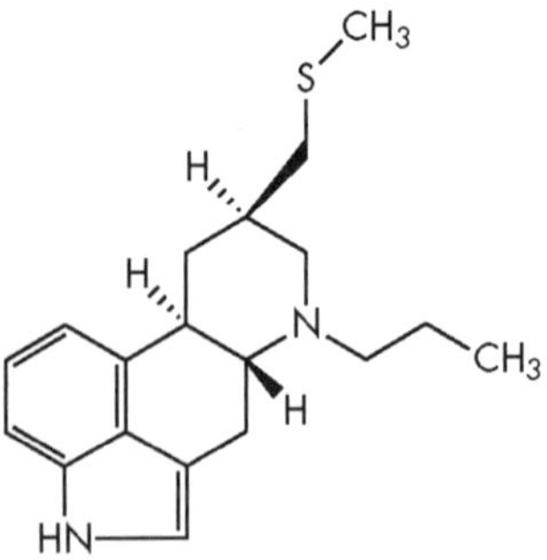

Figure 3.7   Pergolide.

FOCUS ON DOPAMINE AGONISTS 3.8

Pergolide

Dosage

- *Monotherapy:*
  - to initiate therapy:

Day(s)	Morning dose	Midday dose	Evening dose
1	–	–	50 μg
2 to 4	–	50 μg	50 μg
5 to 7	50 μg	50 μg	100 μg
8 to 10	100 μg	100 μg	100 μg
11 to 13	100 μg	150 μg	150 μg
14 to 17	200 μg	200 μg	200 μg
18 to 21	250 μg	250 μg	250 μg
22 to 24	500 μg	250 μg	250 μg
25 to 27	500 μg	500 μg	250 μg
28 to 30	500 μg	500 μg	500 μg

  - after day 30, the daily dose can be increased by up to 250 μg twice a week until the patient achieves optimal therapeutic effect
  - usual maintenance dose is 2–2.5 mg daily in three divided doses
  - maximum dose is 5 mg daily in three divided doses
- *Adjunctive therapy:*
  - initially 50 μg daily for 2 days
  - then increase by 100–150 μg every 3 days for the next 12 days (given in three daily divided doses)
  - the further increases in dosage can be made of 250 μg every 3 days
  - usual maintenance dose is 3 mg daily (given in three daily divided doses)
  - maximum dose is 5 mg daily (given in three divided doses)

Notes

- *Levodopa dosage*: during pergolide titration, the dosage of levodopa may be cautiously reduced.
- *Stopping treatment*: when stopping dopamine agonist therapy, this should be done gradually.

Preparations

- Tablets of 50 μg pergolide (as mesilate) (Celance)
- Tablets of 250 μg pergolide (as mesilate) (Celance)
- Tablets of 1 mg pergolide (as mesilate) (Celance)

Note: also available as a non-proprietary product.

Side-effects
See also under Ergot derivatives and Bromocriptine.

The most commonly reported side-effects with pergolide are nausea, vomiting, dyspepsia, abdominal pain, dyskinesia, hallucinations and confusion. Recent studies have shown that pergolide can have adverse effects on the heart, resulting in a cardiac vulvulopathy.[8] This, together with the potential toxic effects associated with ergot derivatives, has increased reluctance to use pergolide. If it is used, regular echocardiograms should be performed and the drug stopped if cardiac effects are identified.

Interactions
See Bromocriptine.

Pharmacokinetics
After absorption from the gastrointestinal tract, pergolide is extensively metabolised. Some of the metabolites might have dopamine agonist activity. The kidney is the major route of excretion. Pergolide is approximately 90% bound to plasma proteins.

See Focus on dopamine agonists (3.8).

Non-ergot derivative dopamine agonists

Pramipexole and ropinirole are dopamine agonists that are not derivatives of ergot. They are used as monotherapy as well as adjunctive therapy with levodopa. These newer agents do not cause the serious fibrotic reactions that have been associated with the use of the older ergot-derived compounds. For this reason they are the preferred dopamine agonists and often used in younger patients. Although not quite as effective as levodopa, pramipexole and ropinirole produce fewer problems with dyskinesia, the wearing-off phenomenon and 'on/off' motor fluctuations that are often a problem with levodopa therapy.

Pramipexole

Pramipexole (see Figure 3.8) has a greater affinity for D_3 receptors than the other dopamine agonists. Whether this imparts any advantage in the pharmacology of the drug is not known.

Side-effects
Some of the side-effects such as somnolence are dependent on the dosage used. Somnolence is much more likely to be a problem with doses of

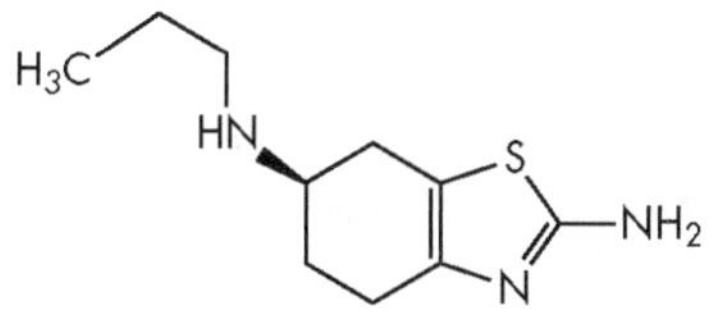

Figure 3.8 Pramipexole.

more than 1.05 mg daily (expressed as base). Common side-effects including constipation, nausea and dyskinesia are often transient. Postural hypotension can normally by avoided by increasing the dosage of pramipexole gradually. As with other drugs in this group, insomnia, hallucinations and confusion can be troublesome. Peripheral oedema can also occur.

Dopamine agonists have been implicated in causing pathological gambling.[9] The cause of this is unknown, but evidence is strong that these drugs precipitate this behaviour. The pathological gambling is reversible and the problem resolves on stopping the dopamine agonist. Pramipexole seems to have a higher risk of causing pathological gambling. It has been suggested this relates to a disproportionate stimulation of dopamine D_3 receptors.

Interactions
Potential interactions are similar to those for bromocriptine (see page 44). Additionally, the renal clearance of pramipexole can be reduced by approximately one-third following concomitant administration of cimetidine. This can significantly increase pramipexole plasma levels necessitating a reduction in dosage.

Pharmacokinetics
Following oral administration, pramipexole is rapidly and completely absorbed. Peak blood levels occur between one and three hours and bioavailability is in the region of 90%. Although food does not reduce the amount of drug absorbed, the rate of absorption is decreased. Pramipexole is only 20% protein bound. It readily passes into the central nervous system; animal studies have shown concentrations in brain reach eight times those in blood. Very little of the drug is metabolised and it is largely excreted unchanged in the urine. The elimination half-life ranges from 8 h to 12 h.

See Focus on dopamine agonists (3.9).

FOCUS ON DOPAMINE AGONISTS 3.9

Pramipexole

Dosage

NB: the dosages below are expressed in terms of milligrams of base.

- Week 1: 88 μg three times daily
- Week 2: 180 μg three times daily
- Week 3: 350 μg times daily
- Thereafter:
    - increase daily dose by 0.75 mg at weekly intervals if necessary to achieve maximal therapeutic effect, providing the patient does not experience unacceptable side-effects
    - maximum daily dose is 3.3 mg in individual doses.

Notes

- *Adjunctive therapy to levodopa*: the dosage of levodopa may need to be reduced during titration and maintenance treatment with pramipexole.
- *Food*: doses may be taken with or without food.
- *Stopping treatment*: when stopping dopamine agonist therapy, this should be done gradually.

Preparations

NB: 1 mg of pramipexole dihydrochloride monohydrate (salt) is equivalent to 0.7 mg of pramipexole base.

Tablet strengths:

- 88 μg (expressed as base) of pramipexole dihydrochloride monohydrate (Mirapexin)
- 180 μg (expressed as base) of pramipexole dihydrochloride monohydrate (Mirapexin)
- 700 μg (expressed as base) of pramipexole dihydrochloride monohydrate (Mirapexin)
- It is planned that a 350 μg (expressed as base) tablet will become available in the UK shortly

---

Ropinirole

Ropinirole (see Figure 3.9) is a non-ergot-derived dopamine agonist similar to pramipexole. A long-term study has recently been presented which suggests that dyskinesia is substantially less when patients are initially started on ropinirole and levodopa added in when symptoms necessitate, compared to the extent of dykinesia experienced when

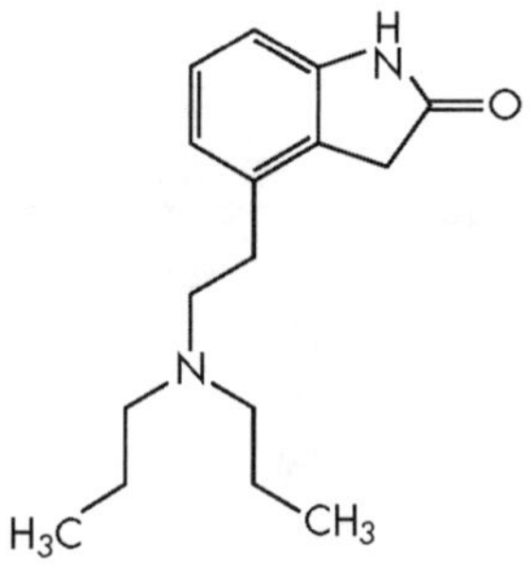

Figure 3.9 Ropinirole.

levodopa is used as the initial treatment.[10] Results at ten years showed that the incidence of dyskinesia was approximately 80% in patients who were initiated with levodopa, and 50% in those patients who commenced therapy with ropinirole. The mean time to the occurrence of dyskinesia was increased by more than 18 months in patients starting with ropinirole therapy. Although these results are encouraging, criticism of the study design casts a degree of doubt on their validity.

Side-effects
The side-effect profile of ropinirole is similar to that of pramipexole. Somnolence, nausea, vomiting and oedema are the problems most frequently encountered. There is some evidence that ropinirole causes less postural hypotension than some of the other dopamine agonists. However, this side-effect does occur in some patients and can be severe. Dyskinesia, hallucinations and confusion are more noticeable when ropinirole is used as adjunctive therapy with levodopa.

Interactions
Potential interaction are similar to those for bromocriptine (see page 44).

The plasma concentration of ropinirole may be increased in patients treated with high doses of oestrogens. If the dosage of ropinirole is titrated to achieve optimal control of symptoms while the patient is on hormone replacement therapy (HRT), an adjustment in dosage may be necessary if HRT is stopped. If HRT is commenced in a patient who is on a maintenance dose of ropinirole, again, the dosage may need to be adjusted.

FOCUS ON DOPAMINE AGONISTS 3.10

Ropinirole

Dosage

- Week 1: 0.25 mg three times daily
- Week 2: 0.5 mg three times daily
- Week 3: 0.75 mg three times daily
- Week 4: 1 mg three times daily
- Thereafter:
  - dosage may be increased at weekly intervals by up to 3 mg per day if necessary to achieve maximal therapeutic effect, providing the patient does not experience unacceptable side-effects
  - maximum daily dose is 24 mg

Notes

- *Adjunctive therapy to levodopa*: when used at adjunctive therapy with levodopa, the dosage of levodopa may be gradually reduced by approximately 20%.
- *Food*: doses should be taken with meals to reduce the likelihood of gastrointestinal side-effects.
- *Stopping treatment*: when stopping dopamine agonist therapy, this should be done gradually.

Preparations

Tablet strengths:

- 0.25 mg ropinirole (as hydrochloride) (Requip)
- 0.5 mg ropinirole (as hydrochloride) (Requip)
- 1 mg ropinerole (as hydrochloride) (Requip)
- 2 mg ropinirole (as hydrochloride) (Requip)
- 5 mg ropinirole (as hydrochloride) (Requip)

Note: for initiating treatment, a starter-pack is available to facilitate dose escalation (containing 42 × 0.25 mg tablets; 42 × 0.5 mg tablets; 21 × 1 mg tablets). A follow-on pack is also available if further escalation in dosage is required (containing 42 × 0.5 mg tablets; 42 × 1 mg tablets; 63 × 2 mg tablets).

Pharmacokinetics

The absorption of ropinirole from the gastrointestinal tract is rapid and almost complete. Peak levels in the blood occur after approximately 1.5 h. There is some evidence that the rate of absorption may be reduced if the drug is taken with food; however, the total amount absorbed remains unaffected. The binding of ropinirole to plasma proteins is low

(10–40%). It is metabolised in the liver, primarily by oxidative metabolism, and the metabolites excreted in the urine.

See Focus on dopamine agonists (3.10).

Apomorphine

Apomorphine (see Figure 3.10) is a very potent dopamine agonist which
stimulates both the D_1 and D_2 groups of receptors. It was first used as
a treatment for Parkinson's disease in 1951, but it was not until much
later when a way was found to block its potent emetic properties that
it became an acceptable treatment option. It is administered by the
subcutaneous route to avoid extensive first-pass liver metabolism which
produces an inactive metabolite. Various other routes of administration
have been tried including intranasal, transdermal and sublingual, but so
far these have proved to be less effective and at present subcutaneous
injections or continuous subcutaneous infusion are the only methods
available for administering the drug in clinical practice. Results of a
phase II study of inhaled apomorphine which were released in the
summer of 2006 are a little more encouraging.[11] Conducted in 24
patients with Parkinson's disease, the drug was administered after an
'off' episode was induced. Just over one-half of the patients receiving
active drug converted from the 'off' state, and one-half of these successfully achieved a full 'on' state. Onset of therapeutic effect took approximately 10 min and lasted about 25 min. Apomorphine is useful as a
diagnostic tool since it has a rapid onset of action of between 5 and
15 min. Its beneficial effects last for approximately 1 h. When used as
treatment it can be given either as rescue therapy (similar to its use as a
diagnostic tool) or as a subcutaneous infusion via a small portable
pump. It is mainly used in patients who experience disabling 'on/off'
motor fluctuations or have severe problems with peak-dose dyskinesias
from levodopa therapy. Patients who are reasonably well during 'on'
times, but suffer badly during 'off' periods tend to benefit most from
treatment with apomorphine.

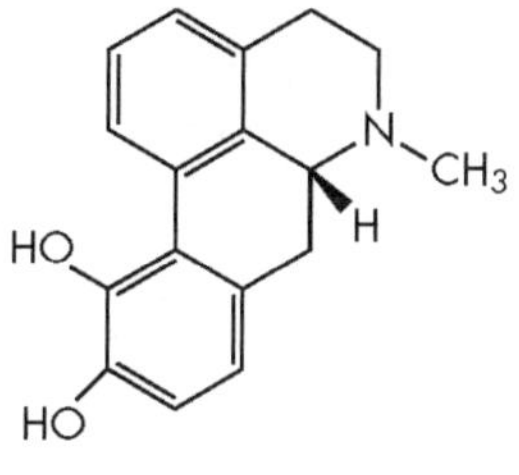

Figure 3.10   Apomorphine.

Commencing treatment

The dose of apomorphine needs to be carefully titrated according to an individual's response to the drug and the appearance of side-effects. This is usually done within a hospital with neurological expertise, normally as an inpatient, occasionally as a day patient.

An apomorphine challenge is used to confirm the drug produces a useful therapeutic effect in the patient and to establish the likely dosage that will be necessary, as well as identifying side-effects that may occur, especially postural hypotension and hallucinations. In order to counter the emetic effects of apomorphine, domperidone at a dose of 20 mg three times daily is started 72 h prior to the administration of apomorphine. Existing anti-Parkinson's drug therapy is stopped 4–6 h before the scheduled time for receiving the apomorphine. This will result in an 'off' state enabling the therapeutic effects of apomorphine to be ascertained. A rating scale is used to assess motor function prior to administering a 1 mg dose of apomorphine. Assessment is repeated during the following 30 min and the patient observed for the occurrence of any side-effects. After this time if little or no response is seen, a further dose of 3 mg can be given and further assessment carried out. Again, further doses (5 mg and 7 mg) can be given at 30 min intervals until a response is seen or a dosage of 7 mg has been reached. If no response is observed on administering 7 mg, the patient is considered a non-responder. In some cases, if a small degree of response is seen at 7 mg, a dose of 10 mg can be given.

Intermittent injections

In patients who obtain a beneficial response to apomorphine, intermittent injections can be used as 'rescue' from severe 'off' periods. Oral therapy is still maintained and should be optimised to keep the needs for rescue to a minimum. Clearly, the injection needs to be given at the onset of symptoms, or when the patient 'senses' an impending 'off' period, which many do. Failing to give the injection at this time will mean administration becomes very difficult once severe symptoms develop. A prefilled, multidose pen (APO-go Pen) is available and is designed to be unobtrusive and make injections as easy as possible (see Plate 7).

Continuous infusion

For patients requiring frequent injections (more than six per day), a continuous subcutaneous infusion delivering the drug during waking hours may provide an alternative option. A small portable syringe driver specifically designed to enable the dose rate and size of bolus doses to be accurately set is used (APO-go Pump). This device is compact and lightweight, and features a display giving details of the settings and providing information to the patient on the length of infusion remaining (see Plates 7 and 8). Prefilled syringes are supplied to the patient, who is trained to connect these to the syringe driver and insert the cannula delivering the drug subcutaneously, usually in the anterior abdominal wall or the outer aspects of the thigh. It is important that patients rotate the location of the injection site to reduce the risk of excessive irritation and nodule formation.

Britannia Pharmaceuticals, who market apomorphine injection in the UK, supply the infusion pump on a loan basis free of charge to the patient. They also have a website which provides further information and support to patients using apomorphine.

Side-effects

The nausea and vomiting caused by apomorphine are effectively prevented by concurrent administration of domperidone. This is the anti-emetic of choice since others such as metoclopramide cross the blood–brain barrier and may cause central effects exacerbating the symptoms of Parkinson's disease. They may also directly interact with certain anti-Parkinson's drugs. Some patients find that after a few months of treatment with apomorphine, an anti-emetic is no longer necessary. Hallucinations and mental confusion can occur and may limit the dosage that can be administered. Postural hypotension can also be troublesome. Local reactions at the sites of injection are more common with infusion than intermittent injections. Sometimes nodules develop under the skin which may be treated with ultrasound (see Plate 8). Occasionally these nodules become infected and antibiotic therapy becomes necessary. Attention to good skin hygiene reduces this risk.

See Focus on Dopamine agonists (3.11).

Rotigotine

Rotigotine (see Figure 3.11) was launched in the UK during the early part of 2006 and was the first agent formulated for transdermal delivery from a patch applied to the skin to become generally available for clinical use. This may improve convenience for the patient as a new patch is applied just once a day, but in addition to this advantage, the transdermal patch delivers a constant supply of drug resulting in continuous stimulation of the dopamine receptors in the brain. This more closely mimics the normal physiological situation which is

FOCUS ON DOPAMINE AGONISTS 3.11

Apomorphine

Dosage

- *Subcutaneous injection:*
  - dosage is individualised to patient needs and tolerance to the drug, but is usually within the range of 3–30 mg daily in divided doses
  - maximum single dose is 10 mg
- *Subcutaneous infusion:*
  - initially 1 mg/h
  - increased according to response and tolerance to the drug in increments of 500 µg/h
  - maximum infusion rate is 4 mg/h

Notes

- *Subcutaneous infusion:*
  - the infusion site should be changed every 12 h
  - in some patients bolus doses may be administered intermittently.
- *Subcutaneous injection and subcutaneous infusion*: total daily maximum dose by all routes is 100 mg.

Preparations

- Injections of apomorphine (APO-go)
  - Ampoules: 10 mg per ml, 2 ml and 5 ml ampoules
  - APO-go Pen: 10 mg per ml, 3 ml pen injector

considered necessary to avoid the onset of dyskinesia. There is evidence that pulsatile stimulation of dopamine receptors produces postsynaptic changes in the striatal neurons. These changes seem to affect nearby glutamate receptors causing overactivity. This ultimately results in some of the long-term problems that develop, such as dyskinesia and 'on/off' motor fluctuations. Until now, the only methods available for achieving continuous stimulation with dopamine agonists have been continuous subcutaneous infusions of apomorphine and the use of cabergoline which has a very long half-life of 65 h. Levodopa can also be administered continuously, as a gel via an intra-duodenal pump, but as with the continuous apomorphine infusion, the method is not straightforward and is certainly more cumbersome than applying a small patch to the skin. A further advantage is that transdermal treatment avoids first-pass hepatic metabolism and potential problems with absorption from the gastrointestinal tract. Both of these factors can substantially influence

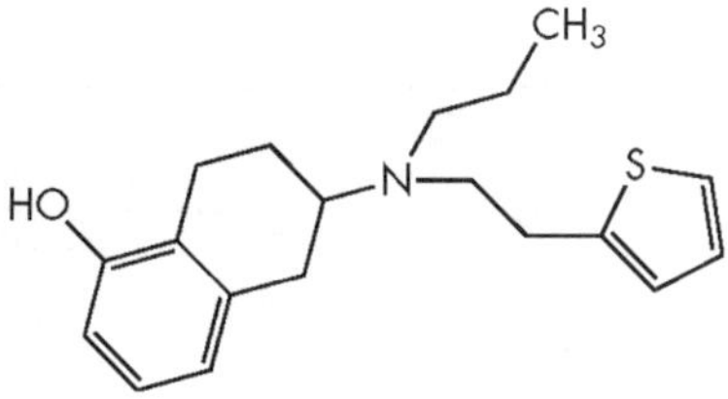

Figure 3.11   Rotigotine.

the bioavailability of drugs used in the treatment of Parkinson's disease and lead to significant variations in the control of symptoms. Dysphagia is often a problem associated with Parkinson's disease, and transdermal patches may provide a way of reducing the number of tablets that have to be swallowed.

Rotigotine is not related to ergot and is not therefore liable to cause serious adverse effects such as fibrotic reactions. It is a selective agonist of dopamine D_2 receptors, but also possesses 5-hydroxytryptamine 1A agonist and α_2-adrenergic antagonist properties. Rotigotine is lipid soluble and penetrates the skin producing therapeutic levels systemically. At the time of writing, only placebo-controlled studies were found, but these clearly demonstrate a useful clinical effect. A trial carried out assessing the benefits of rotigotine treatment after 11 weeks showed improvements in a number of outcome measures.[12] Amongst other adverse effects, two patients in this trial experienced serious effects while driving that were attributed to the drug. The first had an episode of sudden onset of sleep, the other had a brief loss of consciousness. A more recent study was of longer duration and confirmed the therapeutic effects at 27 weeks.[13] In both studies, local site reactions occurred in approximately half of patients using rotigotine patches.

Adverse effects
In addition to the local reactions where the patch has been applied, nausea and vomiting may occur. These are particularly troublesome in the early days of treatment, but if the patient perseveres, these unwanted effects are usually transient. Patients may experience dizziness, headache, somnolence, hallucinations, orthostatic hypotension and fatigue. Effects on the gastrointestinal tract include constipation, diarrhoea and dyspepsia. Sudden onset of sleep is obviously a serious problem and can occur with a number of drugs used to treat Parkinson's disease. Less common side-effects include decreased appetite, visual disturbances, palpitations, and skin reactions.

FOCUS ON DOPAMINE AGONISTS 3.12

Rotigotine

Dosage

- Applied as a transdermal patch:
  - week 1: 2 mg per 24 h
  - week 2: 4 mg per 24 h
  - some patients find this an effective dose and no further increases are necessary
- If inadequate response is achieved:
  - week 3: 6 mg per 24 h
  - some patients find this an effective dose and no further increases are necessary
- If inadequate response is achieved:
  - week 4: 8 mg per 24 h
- Most patients require 6 mg per 24 h or 8 mg per 24 h for effective treatment
- The maximum dose is 8 mg per 24 h

Notes

- *Application of patches:*
  - a patch is applied at approximately the same time each day
  - the patch is normally left on for the full 24 h period
  - sites of application should be rotated; re-application to the same site should be avoided for 2 weeks
  - the patch should be applied to clean, dry, intact healthy skin
  - the recommended sites for application are: abdomen, thigh, hip, flank, shoulder or upper arm.
- *Stopping treatment:* treatment with rotigotine patches should be stopped gradually. This is done by decreasing the dosage on alternate days by using the next lowest strength of patch.

Preparations

There are four strengths of rotigotine transdermal patches (Neupro):

- 2 mg per 24 h (each patch of 10 cm^2 contains 4.5 mg of rotigotine)
- 4 mg per 24 h (each patch of 20 cm^2 contains 9.0 mg of rotigotine)
- 6 mg per 24 h (each patch of 30 cm^2 contains 13.5 mg of rotigotine)
- 8 mg per 24 h (each patch of 40 cm^2 contains 18.0 mg of rotigotine).

Note: an initiation pack containing 28 patches is available (seven patches each of: 2, 4, 6 and 8 mg per 24 h).

Interactions

Although firm evidence is lacking, it is assumed that drugs which are dopamine antagonists such as phenothiazines, butyrophenones, thioxanthines and metoclopramide may reduce the effectiveness of rotigotine. Other drugs that have CNS-depressant effects, including alcohol, are likely to increase the risk of some side-effects. Rotigotine is licensed for use as monotherapy and as combination therapy with levodopa; in the latter case it has the potential to increase the dopaminergic side-effects of levodopa and precipitate or exacerbate dyskinesia.

Pharmacokinetics

Rotigotine is absorbed through the skin and steady-state concentrations are achieved after 1 or 2 days of using the transdermal patches. *In vitro* data suggest that the drug is 92% bound to plasma proteins. Rotigotine is mainly metabolised by N-dealkylation and then conjugation to form sulphates and glucuronides. These metabolites are primarily excreted in the urine.

See Focus on dopamine agonists (3.12).

Anticholinergic drugs

The poisonous plant commonly known as deadly nightshade (*Atropa belladonna*) provided the first effective treatment for patients suffering with Parkinson's disease. The leaves and other parts contain a number of antimuscarinic alkaloids including hyoscyamine (the levo-isomer of atropine) and hyoscine (scopolamine). In the late 1800s, belladonna was introduced and provided for the first time a therapy that produced useful benefit in some who suffered with Parkinson's disease. These days the use of anticholinergic agents to treat Parkinson's disease is somewhat limited, and on the occasions that this pharmacological approach is deployed, synthetic compounds rather than leaves of deadly nightshade are preferred!

The early-day model used to describe what goes wrong in Parkinson's disease and how drugs produce a useful effect consists of a push–pull mechanism between acetylcholine and dopamine in the corpus striatum (see Figure 2.3, page 16). The acetylcholine has a stimulatory effect on nerve cells, while dopamine has an inhibitory effect. When in balance, normal control of movement is possible, but when less dopamine is available as a result of Parkinson's disease, the balance is lost resulting in the motor symptoms of the disease. Although far from being an accurate model of the mechanism, it does offer a way of envisaging how restoring the balance by increasing the level of dopamine can reduce symptoms. Equally, it is possible to use the model to explain how blocking the effects of acetylcholine restores the balance between the two neurotransmitters. The anticholinergic drugs do produce improvement in some symptoms of Parkinson's disease, but these days more effective drugs which are also better tolerated are used in the majority of patients.

Anticholinergic drugs have little effect on symptoms such as hypokinesia and bradykinesia, or rigidity. However, they can dramatically improve the tremor associated with Parkinson's disease. In patients where this is the most troublesome symptom, anticholinergics still have a place. This form of treatment may be more effective than levodopa in treating severe tremor and dystonia. Although the use of these drugs in Parkinson's disease is somewhat limited, they are effective in the treatment of drug-induced parkinsonism. Adverse effects associated with the use of anticholinergic drugs are a major problem. This limits their use and the dosage that can be used to achieve the desired improvement in symptoms. Although the newer compounds have fewer peripheral problems than the older drugs such as hyoscine, these unwanted anticholinergic effects can be very significant and include dry mouth, constipation, blurred vision and urinary retention. Central effects such as confusion, restlessness, hallucinations and euphoria can also be severe.

Trihexphenidyl (see Figure 3.12) (formerly known as benzhexol) and orphenadrine (see Figure 3.13) are the drugs that are still occasionally used in Parkinson's disease. Procyclidine (see Figure 3.14) and benztropine (only available as an injection) are mainly used for treating drug-induced extrapyramidal symptoms. Details of dosage and preparations available for trihexyphenidyl, orphenadrine and procyclidine are given in Focus on anticholinergic drugs (3.13).

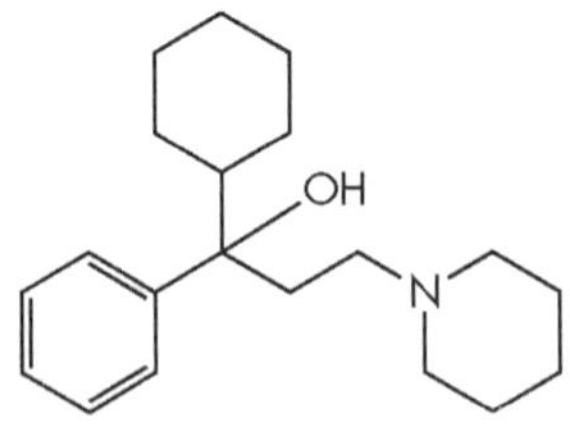

Figure 3.12 Trihexyphenidyl.

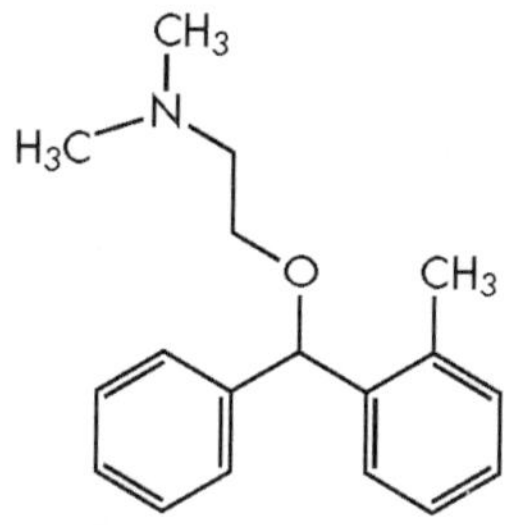

Figure 3.13   Orphenadrine.

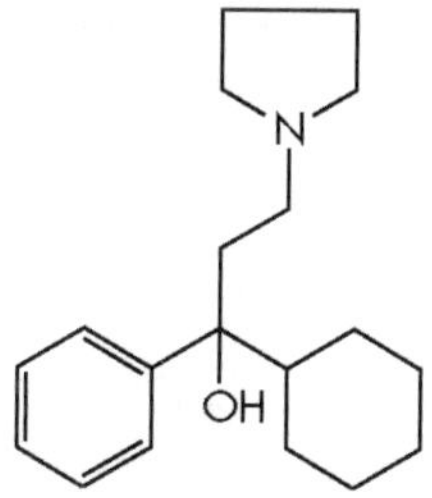

Figure 3.14   Procyclidine.

FOCUS ON ANTICHOLINERGIC DRUGS 3.13

Trihexphenidyl (formerly called benzhexol)

Dosage

- Initially 1 mg daily gradually increased according to response and adverse effects
- Usual maintenance dose is 5–15 mg daily in three or four divided doses
- Maximum dose is 20 mg daily in three or four divided doses

Notes

- *Food*: doses should be taken before or after food.
- *Elderly patients*: adverse effects are more likely to occur and therefore the dosage should be increased slowly and the total amount taken each day kept to a minimum.
- *Driving*: the ability to perform skilled tasks may be impaired.

Preparations

- Trihexphenidyl hydrochloride 2 mg and 5 mg tablets
- Trihexphenidyl hydrochloride (Broflex) 5 mg per 5 ml oral liquid

continued overleaf

Focus on anticholinergic drugs 3.13 (continued)

Orphenadrine

Dosage

- Initially 150 mg daily in divided doses gradually increased according to response and adverse effects
- Maximum dose is 400 mg daily in three or four divided doses

Notes

- *Elderly patients*: adverse effects are more likely to occur and therefore the dosage should be increased slowly and the total amount taken each day kept to a minimum.
- *Driving*: the ability to perform skilled tasks may be impaired.

Preparations

- Orphenadrine hydrochloride (Disipal) 50 mg tablets
- Orphenadrine hydrochloride (Biorphen) 25 mg per 5 ml oral liquid
- Orphenadrine hydrochloride (non-proprietary) 50 mg per 5 ml oral liquid
- Orphenadrine hydrochloride tablets are also available as a non-proprietary product

Procyclidine

Dosage

- Initially 2.5 mg three times daily gradually increased according to response and adverse effects
- Maximum dose is usually 10 mg three times daily

Notes

- *Elderly patients*: adverse effects are more likely to occur and therefore the dosage should be increased slowly and the total amount taken each day kept to a minimum.
- *Driving*: the ability to perform skilled tasks may be impaired.

Preparations

- Procyclidine hydrochloride (Kemadrin) 5 mg tablets
- Procyclidine hydrochloride (Arpicolin) 2.5 mg per 5 ml, and 5 mg per 5 ml oral liquid
- Procyclidine hydrochloride (Kemadrin) 10 mg per 2 ml ampoules
- Procyclidine hydrochloride tablets are also available as a non-proprietary product

Monoamine oxidase-B inhibitors

Monoamine oxidase (MAO) is an enzyme that inactivates dopamine, reducing the levels available to facilitate transmission in the dopaminergic pathways. Administration of an inhibitor of MAO blocks this breakdown in neurons and glial cells in the brain, increasing the amount of dopamine available in the striatum for synaptic transmission. Early inhibitors of MAO were introduced in the 1950s to treat depression, and in the 1960s were assessed for their value in treating Parkinson's disease. Not only were the results disappointing, but the potential hazards of the severe reactions produced when these MAO inhibitors were taken with certain foods and other drugs presented a major risk. Foods rich in tyramine such as mature cheese, pickled herring, broad bean pods, meat and yeast extracts, and fish, poultry and meat that is not fresh can cause a serious increase in blood pressure when taken with these initial MAO inhibitors. Similarly a number of drugs such as sympathomimetics can interact, resulting in hypertensive crisis. The danger of such interactions remains for up to 2 weeks after stopping the MAO inhibitor. Later work led to the discovery of two types of MAO inhibitor, type A and type B. MAO-B inhibitors were found not to cause these serious reactions resulting from interaction with other drugs or foods. It is the type B inhibitor which subsequently became part of the portfolio of drugs used for treating Parkinson's disease. Two are now available, selegiline and rasagiline.

Selegiline

In the 1970s, selegiline (see Figure 3.15) was introduced and found to have a useful effect, albeit modest, on the symptoms of Parkinson's disease. Its main use has been in the early stages of the disease when symptoms are very mild, and as an adjunct to levodopa especially to reduce problems with the end-of-dose wearing-off effect. For many years there has been a disputed claim that selegiline has a delaying effect on disease progression. Evidence for such an effect is very poor. Its ability to reduce free radical formation has been offered as a mechanism, and some data from clinical studies have been interpreted suggesting an effect on progression of Parkinson's disease.

The results from the DATATOP study (Deprenyl and Tocopherol Antioxidative Therapy of Parkinsonism) showed that selegiline significantly delayed the need to start levodopa therapy in previously untreated patients.[14] Subjects in this blinded, randomised trial were given either placebo, deprenyl (selegiline) or tocopherol (a component of vitamin E).

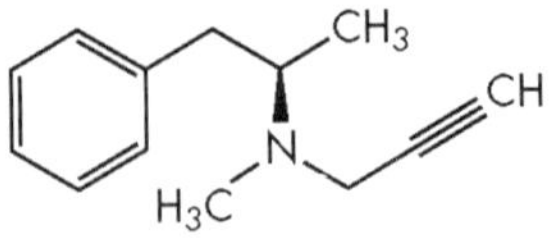

Figure 3.15   Selegiline.

The results at 12 months showed that selegiline delayed the need for levodopa therapy to be commenced by approximately 9 months. Tocopherol was not found to have any useful effect. Some claim that the effect seen with selegiline is indicative of a neuroprotective effect, others that it was simply the result of better symptom control compared to placebo. A subsequent trial carried out in the UK however produced major concerns when an increase in mortality was found in patients receiving levodopa with selegiline, compared to those taking levodopa on its own.[15]

Much debate took place over subsequent years, many criticising the suggestion that selegiline increased the risk of mortality. Since then, several studies have failed to demonstrate an increase in mortality, including a meta-analysis of five randomised, double-blind trials.[16] Controversy persists up to the present time, though the usage of selegiline has picked up again slightly in recent years.

A meta-analysis published in 2004 looked at both the benefits and risks of MAO-B inhibitors in early Parkinson's disease.[17] Seventeen randomised trials were included in the analysis which showed there was no significant difference in mortality between patients receiving MAO-B inhibitors and control patients. The meta-analysis also demonstrated that MAO-B inhibitors reduced disability, with better scores for motor function and activities of daily living compared with the results in patients taking placebo.

Side-effects

Selegiline is generally well tolerated, but can itself cause many of the side-effects that result from levodopa therapy. These include postural hypotension, nausea, dry mouth, sleeping disorders, confusion and hallucinations. An increase in dyskinesias may occur, especially when used as adjunctive therapy with levodopa.

Interactions

Interactions which are well documented with MAO-A inhibitors are unlikely to occur with selegiline due to its selectivity for inhibiting

MAO-B, however, life-threatening interactions can occur with pethidine, tricyclic antidepressants and selective serotonin reuptake inhibitors (SSRIs). It is recommended that starting treatment with selegiline be delayed for at least 5 weeks after stopping previous therapy with fluoxetine. Caution is also advised when tramadol is taken concomitantly. In patients taking a COMT inhibitor (entacapone or tolcapone), the dose of selegiline should not exceed 10 mg daily of the standard formulation.

Pharmacokinetics

Selegiline is rapidly absorbed after oral administration, peak blood levels occurring within 30 min. However, bioavailability is low, typically only one-tenth of the dose taken reaching the systemic circulation when taken as standard formulation tablets, since the drug undergoes extensive first-pass metabolism. Selegiline passes readily into the brain and penetrates tissues peripherally. Between 75% and 85% is bound to plasma proteins. A number of metabolites are produced by the liver including l-amfetamine and l-methamfetamine. These and other metabolites are excreted in the urine. The amfetamine metabolites may cause insomnia and abnormal dreams. It is therefore recommended that doses are not taken late in the day. The dose of drug absorbed from the tongue when the freeze-dried tablets are used does not produce the same concentrations of amfetamine metabolites, these being reduced by approximately 90%.

Rasagiline

During 2005, rasagiline (see Figure 3.16) became available. This, like selegiline, is a selective MAO-B inhibitor and is only the second drug with this pharmacological action to be introduced in the UK for the treatment of Parkinson's disease. It can be used as monotherapy or as adjunctive therapy with co-careldopa or co-beneldopa in those patients suffering with end-of-dose fluctuations. Since the main pharmacological properties of rasagiline are the same as those of selegiline, it shares many of this drug's side-effects and potential interactions. Since no comparative studies have been carried out between the two drugs it is difficult at this stage to assess any differences there might be, either in terms of problems with treatment or clinical benefit. One study has compared the effects of rasagiline with those of the COMT inhibitor entacapone when used as adjunctive treatment with levodopa plus decarboxylase inhibitor. This showed that these two drugs have a similar effect on 'off' time (see page 68).

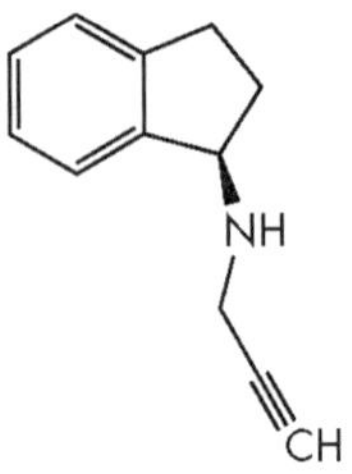

Figure 3.16 Rasagiline.

A series of papers have been published which seem to have been orchestrated with a musical theme in mind:

- TEMPO (TVP-1012 in Early Monotherapy for Parkinson's disease Outpatients)
- LARGO (Lasting effect in Adjunctive therapy with Rasagiline Given Once daily)
- PRESTO (Parkinson's Rasagiline: Efficacy and Safety in the Treatment of Off).

The TEMPO study was carried out in over 400 patients with early Parkinson's disease.[18] Monotherapy with rasagiline 1 mg or 2 mg or placebo was given for 26 weeks. Improvements were seen in the motor subscale of the UPDRS and the activities of daily living subscale. At the end of the 26-week period, all patients continued treatment with 2 mg rasagiline for a further 6 months. Analysis of the results showed a smaller increase in UPDRS in patients who had received active drug for the whole year compared to those who had only received rasagiline for 6 months. It has been suggested this indicates that starting treatment at an early stage of the disease reduces functional decline.[19] However much more work needs to be carried out before any claims that the drug decreases disease progression are proven.

The LARGO study was carried out in 687 patients.[20] Each of three groups received either rasagiline 1 mg, entacapone with levodopa or placebo. The rasagiline and entacapone groups decreased off-time to the same extent (by approximately 1.2 h compared to 24 min for placebo). Dyskinesia-free on-time was increased by approximately 50 min in each of the treatment groups and only by a couple of minutes in patients receiving placebo. UPDRS scores for activities of daily living also showed each of the treatments were better than placebo.

The PRESTO study looked at the effects of rasagiline in 472 patients who were suffering with at least 2.5 h off-time per day.[21]

Existing treatment was optimised before patients were allocated to one of three groups: rasagiline 0.5 mg, rasagiline 1 mg or placebo. After 26 weeks, off-time was decreased by 1.41 h and 1.85 h in the rasagiline 0.5 mg and 1 mg groups respectively. In the placebo group, off-time was reduced by only 0.91 h.

Side-effects

Rasagiline may cause fewer problems with insomnia compared to selegiline when this drug is given in the standard formulation tablet. This can be explained by the lack of amfetamine metabolites produced by rasagiline.

For further information on side-effects, see Selegiline.

Interactions

See Selegiline.

Pharmacokinetics

Rasagiline is absorbed rapidly, producing peak plasma levels in 30 min. About one-third of the dose is bioavailable. Rasagiline can be taken with or without food, though meals that are high in fat can produce a decrease in levels; however, there is only a slight reduction in the total amount absorbed. The drug is 60–70% bound to plasma proteins. Nearly all of the absorbed drug is metabolised in the liver by dealkylation or hydroxylation. Conjugation of rasagiline and its metabolites with glucuronic acid also occurs. Less than 1% of rasagiline is excreted in the urine unchanged.

See Focus on monoamine oxidase inhibitors (3.14).

COMT inhibitors

Although the amount of levodopa available to produce useful effect is substantially increased by blocking its peripheral breakdown when administering with a dopa decarboxylase inhibitor, there are other enzymes that metabolise the drug. COMT metabolises both levodopa and dopamine in the body. Blocking this enzyme with a COMT inhibitor can further increase the availability of levodopa and prolong its therapeutic effect. Some of the problems associated with fluctuation in the levels of levodopa are therefore reduced with this class of drug.

FOCUS ON MAO INHIBITORS 3.14

Selegiline

Dosage

- *Standard formulation*: 10 mg each morning *or* 5 mg at breakfast and 5 mg at midday
- *Freeze-dried formulation (Zelapar)*: initially 1.25 mg each morning before breakfast (see notes below)

Notes

- *Elderly patients*: when using the standard formulation, the dosage is started at 2.5 mg each morning to reduce the risk of confusion and agitation.
- *Freeze-dried formulation (Zelapar)*: tablets of the freeze-dried formulation are allowed to dissolve after placing on the tongue. Patients should not drink or rinse the mouth out until 5 min have lapsed since taking the tablet. Absorption from this route avoids first-pass metabolism. A dose of 10 mg of the standard formulation is equivalent to taking 1.25 mg of the freeze-dried formulation.

Preparations

- *Standard formulation (Eldepryl)*: selegiline 5 mg and 10 mg tablets, and 10 mg per 5 ml oral liquid
- *Freeze-dried formulation (Zelapar)*: selegiline 1.25 mg tablets

---

Rasagiline

Dosage

- 1 mg each day

Preparations

- Rasagiline (Azilect) 1 mg tablets

COMT inhibitors can be an effective adjunct to co-careldopa and co-beneldopa, reducing both the 'off' time experienced by many patients as well as the end-of-dose deterioration. Two COMT inhibitors are currently available, entacapone and tolcapone, though use of the latter is tightly controlled due to concerns about potential toxic effects.

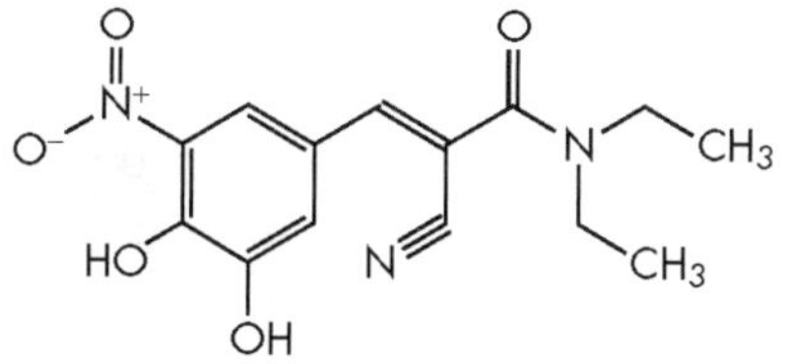

Figure 3.17   Entacapone.

Entacapone

Entacapone (see Figure 3.17) does not cross into the brain and therefore produces its effect by inhibiting COMT peripherally, increasing the bioavailability of levodopa. A dose of 200 mg is taken at the same time as co-careldopa or co-beneldopa, up to a maximum of 2 g daily. It is often necessary to gradually reduce the dosage of levodopa over the first few weeks after starting entacapone. To improve convenience for the patient and reduce the number of tablets that need to be swallowed, entacapone is available as a combination product with co-careldopa. Three combination preparations are available (see Focus on COMT inhibitors 3.15).

Several studies have shown that entacapone reduces motor fluctuations in patients with Parkinson's disease.[22] The 'wearing-off' effect is particularly helped, entacapone increasing on-time by 1.0–1.7 h per day. Other studies suggest that health-related quality-of-life scores can also be improved in patients who do not experience motor fluctuations. It is possible that entacapone given together with levodopa might delay the development of motor fluctuations but this has yet to be shown, although results from animal studies suggest that this may be the case.[23] A study has been carried out to see whether entacapone provides benefit to patients who have a stable response to levodopa and are not experiencing motor complications.[24] No improvement in UPDRS motor scores occurred; however, a range of quality-of-life measures were improved.

Side-effects

Since the bioavailability of levodopa is increased, adverse motor effects and orthostatic hypotension can occur. In most cases this problem can be reduced by decreasing the dosage of levodopa. Other side-effects include nausea, vomiting, constipation, diarrhoea and abdominal pain. Entacapone also produces a red/brown colouration of urine. Patients should be warned of this effect which is harmless. Some patients on entacapone plus levodopa therapy experience drowsiness, and there have been cases of episodes of sudden sleep onset occurring. Patients experiencing these side-effects must not drive or undertake other activities where lack of alertness may be hazardous.

Interactions

The metabolism, and therefore effects, of other drugs which are normally metabolised by COMT may be affected. Such drugs include: apomorphine, methyldopa, dobutamine, dopamine and other sympathomimetics. The absorption of entacapone may be significantly reduced by iron due to chelation. Separating doses of the two drugs by at least 2 h should avoid this interaction. In patients taking selegiline, the dosage should not exceed 10 mg daily if entacapone is being taken as well.

Pharmacokinetics

The absorption of entacapone is not affected by food; however, large variation in absorption occurs between patients and even within the same patient. Entacapone undergoes extensive first-pass metabolism and approximately 35% of an oral dose is absorbed resulting in a peak blood level after about 1 h. Entacapone is rapidly distributed in the body and is extensively bound to plasma proteins. Only 10–20% is excreted in urine, mainly conjugated with glucuronic acid. Most of the dose is excreted in the faeces.

Tolcapone

Tolcapone (see Figure 3.18) acts in a similar way to entacapone, but blocks both peripheral and central COMT. Its side-effects are similar to those of entacapone (see page 71), though additionally it can cause

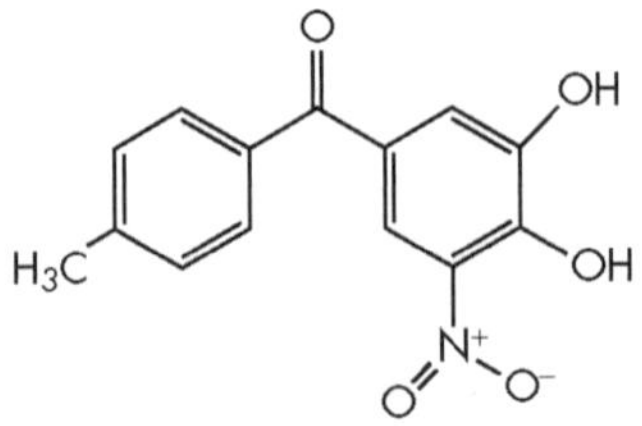

Figure 3.18　Tolcapone.

hepatitis which is potentially fatal. This toxic effect led to the drug being withdrawn from use in the European Union in 1998 after a number of fatalities were attributed to use of the drug. Tolcapone has since become available again, but it should never be used as first-line adjunctive therapy, and strict monitoring is necessary to identify early signs of hepatotoxicity. This includes regular liver function tests every 2 weeks for the first year, every 4 weeks for the next 6 months and then every 8 weeks while the drug is taken. Tolcapone must be stopped if liver function tests, symptoms or signs suggest the onset of liver toxicity. The drug should not be restarted in patients who have previously shown adverse effects on the liver while taking the drug. If tolcapone produces no clinical benefit within 3 weeks of commencing treatment, it should be stopped.

Side-effects

See under Entacapone and discussion above on hepatotoxicity. Tolcapone can produce a harmless yellow colour intensification of urine.

FOCUS ON COMT INHIBITORS 3.15

Entacapone

Dosage

- 200 mg with each dose of levodopa as co-careldopa or co-beneldopa (i.e. levodopa plus peripheral dopa decarboxylase inhibitor)
- Up to a maximum of 2 g daily

Preparations

- Tablets of 200 mg entacapone (Comtess)
- Combination preparations with co-careldopa (Stalevo):

	Levodopa	Carbidopa	Entacapone
Stalevo 50 mg/12.5 mg/200 mg tablets	50 mg	12.5 mg	200 mg
Stalevo 100 mg/25 mg/200 mg tablets	100 mg	25 mg	200 mg
Stalevo 150 mg/37.5 mg/200 mg tablets	150 mg	37.5 mg	200 mg

---

continued overleaf

Focus on COMT inhibitors 3.15 (continued)

Notes

- *Transferring preparations:*
  - If transferring from standard-release co-careldopa or co-beneldopa alone, Stavelo is normally initiated at a dose that provides a similar (or slightly lower) amount of levodopa.
  - When transferring patients suffering with dyskinesia or receiving more than 800 mg of levodopa daily, entacapone should be introduced to existing therapy before transfering to Stalevo. NB: the levodopa dose may need to be reduced by 10–30% initially. This can be dose either by extending the intervals between doses or by decreasing the amount of levodopa taken each time, depending on what suits the patients condition best.
  - In patients who are receiving standard-release co-careldopa or co-beneldopa plus entacapone, Stavelo is normally initiated at a dose that provides a similar (or slightly higher) amount of levodopa.

Tolcapone

Dosage

- 100 mg three times daily
- Up to a maximum of 200 mg three times daily (in exceptional circumstances)
- The first dose of the day should be taken with the first dose of co-careldopa or co-beneldopa

Preparations

- Tablets of 100 mg tolcapone (Tasmar)

Notes

- If the patient is taking more than 600 mg daily of levodopa, this should be reduced (e.g. by 30%) when commencing tolcapone; patients on lower doses of levodopa may also require a reduction in dosage.
- Tablets are film coated and should be swallowed whole since the drug has a bitter taste.

Interactions

See Entacapone.

Pharmacokinetics

Tolcapone is rapidly absorbed, resulting in peak levels at 2 h. Food can delay this and also cause a small decrease in the amount of drug absorbed. Tolcapone is highly protein bound and is nearly completely metabolised by conjugation with glucuronic acid prior to urinary excretion.

Glutamate inhibitors

Amantadine

It was quite by chance in the late 1960s that the useful effects amantadine (see Figure 3.19) has on the symptoms of Parkinson's disease were discovered. Originally introduced into medical practice as an antiviral drug, amantadine was given to a patient who happened to suffer with Parkinson's disease. The patient's motor symptoms improved remarkably and subsequent studies were set up to establish the potential value of amantadine in treating Parkinson's disease. The mechanism by which it relieves symptoms is not clear, but it is now considered likely to result from its glutamate-antagonist properties. Older theories are based on possible effects on the dopaminergic and cholinergic pathways. Amantadine is not as effective as many of the drugs used to treat Parkinson's disease, but in some patients improvements are seen in tremor, rigidity and bradykinesia. For many years, amantadine was mainly used in the early stages of Parkinson's disease before symptoms become more severe making it necessary to turn to much more effective therapy with levodopa. Its modest beneficial effects become inadequate with prolonged treatment. The main role of amantadine nowadays is in reducing dyskinesias induced by levodopa in the later stages of the disease. There is evidence that amantadine can substantially decrease dyskinesias;[25] however, it is uncertain how long this useful effect is maintained. One trial suggests the effects of amantadine are significantly reduced after 8 months.

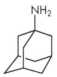

Figure 3.19   Amantadine.

Amantadine interferes with transmission at glutamatergic *N*-methyl-D-aspartate (NMDA) receptors. Animal experiments have shown that this can in turn inhibit the NMDA-evoked release of acetylcholine in striatal tissue. It has also been suggested that amantadine has indirect effects on the nigrostriatal pathway by stimulating dopa decarboxylase activity and the synthesis of dopamine. Positron emission tomography studies have confirmed such an effect in the human brain. More recent research has suggested the glutamate-antagonist properties of amantadine may reduce overactivity of the subthalamic nucleus which may be the cause of dyskinesia. This fits the main therapeutic value of amantadine in clinical practice of reducing drug-induced dyskinesia.

Side-effects

Amantadine can cause a number of side-effects including mental confusion and hallucinations. This is a particular problem in the elderly. If treatment is withdrawn, this should be done slowly, since stopping

FOCUS ON GLUTAMATE INHIBITORS 3.16

Amantadine

Dosage

- Initially 100 mg daily, increased after one week to 100 mg twice daily
- This can be further increased by 100 mg increments up to a maximum of 400 mg daily (see notes below)

Notes

- *Elderly patients*: dosage in the elderly is 100 mg daily, adjusted according to the patient's response.
- *Side-effects*: increasing the dosage increases the likelihood of troublesome side-effects.
- *Withdrawal*: amantadine should be withdrawn gradually by halving the dose at weekly intervals.

Preparations

- Capsules of 100 mg amantadine hydrochloride (Symmetrel)
- Syrup containing 50 mg per 5 ml amantadine hydrochloride (Symmetrel)

Note: the Lysovir brand of amantadine is marketed for the treatment and prophylaxis of influenza A infection.

too rapidly can itself result in acute confusional states. Peripheral oedema and livedo reticularis can also occur in some patients. Insomnia caused by the stimulant effect of the drug can be reduced by avoiding administration after 4 pm.

Interactions

Amantadine increases the risk of extrapyramidal side-effects with a number of drugs including: metoclopramide, domperidone, methyldopa, and antipsychotics. The antimuscarinic side-effects of other drugs may be increased by amantadine.

Pharmacokinetics

The absorption of amantadine from the gastrointestinal tract is nearly 100% and produces peak plasma concentrations within 3–4 h. A substantial proportion of the drug binds to red blood cells; the concentration in erythrocytes is more than 2.5 times that in plasma. It also binds extensively to tissue, the concentrations in organs such as lung, heart, kidney, liver and the spleen being higher than in the blood. Amantadine is mainly excreted unchanged, only a small proportion being excreted as an acetylated metabolite.

See Focus on glutamate inhibitors (3.16).

References

1. Cotzias CG, Van Woert MH, Schiffer LM. Aromatic amino acids and modification of parkinsonism. *N Engl J Med* 1967; 276: 374–379.
2. Fahn S, Oakes D, Shoulson I, *et al.* Levodopa and the progression of Parkinson's disease. *N Engl J Med* 2004; 351: 2498–2508.
3. Nyholm D, Lennernäs H, Gomes-Trolin C, Aquilonius SM. Levodopa pharmacokinetics and motor performance during activities of daily living in patients with Parkinson's disease on individual drug combinations. *Clin Neuropharmacol* 2002; 25: 89–96.
4. Nyholm D, Aquilonius SM. Levodopa infusion therapy in Parkinson's disease: State of the art in 2004. *Clin Neuropharmacol* 2004; 27: 245–256.
5. Nyholm D, Askmark H, Gomes-Trolin C, *et al.* Optimising levodopa pharmacokinetics – intestinal infusion versus oral sustained-release tablets. *Clin Neuropharmacol* 2003; 26: 156–163.
6. Nyholm D, Nilsson Remahl, Dizdar N, *et al.* Duodenal levodopa infusion monotherapy vs oral polypharmacy in advanced Parkinson's disease. *Neurology* 2005; 64: 216–223.
7. Committee on Safety of Medicines. Fibrotic reactions with pergolide and other

ergot-derived dopamine receptor agonists. *Curr Probl Pharmacovigilance* 2002; 28: 3. www.mhra.gov.uk/home/idcplg?IdcService=SS_GET_PAGE&use Secondary=true&ssDocName=CON007453&ssTargetNodeId=368 (accessed 20 June 2007).

8. Van Camp G, Flamez A, Cosyns B, *et al*. Treatment of Parkinson's disease with pergolide and relation to restrictive valvular heart disease. *Lancet* 2004; 363: 1179–1183.

9. Dodd ML, Klos KJ, Bower JH, *et al*. Pathological gambling caused by drugs used to treat Parkinson disease. *Arch Neurol* 2005; 62: 1377–1381.

10. Rascol O, Korczyn AD, De Deyn PP, Lang A. Incidence of dyskinesias in a ten-year naturalistic follow-up of patients with early Parkinson's disease initially receiving ropinirole or L-dopa. Presented at the 16th International Congress on Parkinson's Disease and Related Disorders, Berlin, 2005.

11. Vectura announcement of successful outcome of phase II study on inhaled Parkinson's disease product – VR040. Media release 8 August 2006. www.vectura.com/admin/upload/data/datFiles/press51.asp (accessed 20 June 2007).

12. The Parkinson Study Group. A controlled trial of rotigotine monotherapy in early Parkinson's disease. *Arch Neurol* 2003; 60: 1721–1728.

13. Watts RL, Wendt RL, Nausied B, *et al*. Efficacy, safety and tolerability of the rotigotine transdermal patch in patients with early-stage idiopathic Parkinson's disease: a multicenter, multinational randomised, double-blind trial. *Mov Disord* 2004; 19 (Suppl 9): S258.

14. The Parkinson Study Group. Effect of deprenyl on the progression of disability in early Parkinson's disease. N Engl J Med 1989; 321: 1364–1371.

15. Lees AJ, on behalf of the Parkinson's Disease Research group of the United Kingdom. Comparison of therapeutic effects and mortality data of levodopa and levodopa combined with selegiline in patients with early, mild Parkinson's disease. *BMJ* 1995; 311: 1602–1607.

16. Olanow CW, Myllyla VV, Sotaniemi KA, *et al*. Effects of selegiline on mortality in patients with Parkinson's disease: a meta-analysis. *Neurology* 1998; 51: 825–830.

17. Ives NJ, Stowe RL, Marro J, *et al*. Monoamine oxidase type B inhibitors in early Parkinson's disease: meta-analysis of 17 randomised trials involving 3525 patients. *BMJ* 2004; 329: 593.

18. Parkinson Study Group. A controlled trial of rasagiline in early Parkinson's disease: the TEMPO study. *Arch Neurol* 2002; 59: 1937–1943.

19. Parkinson Study Group. A controlled randomized delayed-start study of rasagiline in early Parkinson disease. *Arch Neurol* 2004; 61: 561–566.

20. Rascol O, Brooks DJ, Melamed E, *et al*. LARGO Study Group. Rasagiline as an adjunct to levodopa in patients with Parkinson's disease and motor fluctuations (LARGO, Lasting effect in Adjunctive therapy with Rasagiline Given Once daily study): a randomised double-blind, parallel-group trial. *Lancet* 2005; 365: 947–954.

21. Parkinson Study Group. A randomised placebo-controlled trial of rasagiline in levodopa-treated patients with Parkinson's disease and motor fluctuations: the PRESTO study. *Arch Neurol* 205; 62: 241–248.

22. Schrag A. Entacapone in the treatment of Parkinson's disease. *Lancet Neurol* 2005; 4: 366–370.

23.   Marin C, Aguilar E, Bonastre M, *et al*. Early administration of entacapone prevents levodopa-induced motor fluctuations in hemiparkinsonian rats. *Exp Neurol* 2005; 192: 184–193.
24.   Olanow CW, Kieburtz K, Stern M, *et al*. Double-blind, placebo-controlled study of entacapone in levodopa-treated patients with stable Parkinson disease. *Arch Neurol* 2004; 61: 1563–1568.
25.   Luginger E, Wenning GK, Bosch S, Poewe W. Beneficial effects of amantadine on L-dopa-induced dyskinesias in Parkinson's disease. *Mov Disord* 2000; 15: 873–878.

Further reading

Brooks DJ, Sagar HJ. Entacapone is beneficial in both fluctuating and non-fluctuating patients with Parkinson's disease. A randomized, placebo-controlled, double-blind six month study. *J Neurol Neurosurg Psychiatry* 2003; 74: 1071–1079.

Chan KL, Jagait P, Tugwell C. Parkinson's disease – current and future aspects of drug treatment. *Hosp Pharm* 2004; 11: 18–22.

Clarke CE. Rasagiline for motor complications in Parkinson's disease. *Lancet* 2005; 365: 914–916.

Crosby NJ, Deane HO, Clarke CE. Amantadine for dyskinesia in Parkinson's disease. (Cochrane Review). *Cochrane Database Syst Rev* 2003; (2): CD003467.

Fahn S, Oakes D, Shoulson I, *et al*. Levodopa and the progression of Parkinson's disease. *N Engl J Med* 2004; 351: 2498–2508.

Holloway RG, Shoulson I, Fahn S, *et al*. Pramipexole vs levodopa as initial treatment for Parkinson disease: a 4-year randomized controlled trial. *Arch Neurol* 2004; 61: 1044–1053.

Navan P, Findley LJ, Undy MB, *et al*. A randomly assigned double-blind cross-over study examining the relative anti-parkinsonian tremor effects of pramipexole and pergolide. *Eur J Neurol* 2005; 12: 1–8.

Nutt JG, Wooten GF. Clinical practice. Diagnosis and initial management of Parkinson's disease. *N Engl J Med* 2005; 353:1021–1027.

Olanow CW, Stocchi F. COMT inhibitors in Parkinson's disease: can they prevent and/or reverse levodopa-induced motor complications? *Neurology* 2004; 62 (Suppl 1): S72–81.

Pahwa R, Factor SA, Lyons KE, *et al*. Practice parameter: treatment of Parkinson disease with motor fluctuations and dyskinesia (an evidence-based review): report of the Quality Standards Subcommittee of the American Academy of Neurology. *Neurology* 2006; 66: 983–995.

Pogarell O, Gasser T, Van Hilten JJ, *et al*. Pramipexole in patients with Parkinson's disease and marked drug resistant tremor: a randomised, double blind, placebo controlled multicentre study. *J Neurol Neurosurg Psychiatry* 2002; 72: 713–720.

Reichmann H, Boas J, Macmahon D, *et al*. Efficacy of combining levodopa with entacapone on quality of life and activities of daily living in patients experiencing wearing-off type fluctuations. *Acta Neurol Scand* 2005; 111: 21–28.

4

Non-drug therapies

Physiotherapy

As with most non-drug therapies used in patients with Parkinson's disease, there is little conclusive evidence in scientific terms that physiotherapy is of significant benefit. However, despite this, many patients, carers and healthcare professionals believe much is gained from physiotherapy, especially in maximising physical mobility and functionality. Not only is the physiotherapy itself of value, but the advice of a physiotherapist on matters such as walking aids, exercise routines, and special techniques to help overcome restrictions in movement, such as getting in and out of bed, can be of great value. Certain forms of physiotherapy such as proprioceptive neuromuscular facilitation (PNF) can help reduce rigidity. PNF is a form of flexibility training which focuses on stretching and contraction of a particular muscle group, increasing the range of movement in patients suffering with rigidity. The Bobath method is used by physiotherapists for a number of neurological conditions including Parkinson's disease. This technique decreases abnormal muscle tone and helps restore more natural movement. It uses inhibiting methods and postures, and involves the physiotherapist utilising specialised handling techniques. Hydrotherapy involves performing exercises in water. These are tailored by the physiotherapist to individual patient needs. In patients with Parkinson's disease, hydrotherapy can enable painful limbs to be moved due to the support given by the buoyancy of the water to weak muscle groups. Moving against the resistance that the water provides helps build up strength in muscles. Hydrotherapy is not the same as swimming, and is suitable for people who cannot swim or have a fear of water. Flotation aids are used for most exercises. Caution needs to be taken with patients who have a tendency to low blood pressure, as can result from some drugs used in Parkinson's disease. The warm water used in hydrotherapy sessions may reduce blood pressure further.

Physiotherapy is often delayed until a patient's symptoms become more disabling. Earlier input by a physiotherapist in providing education and advice may be helpful in maintaining existing fitness and mobility for longer, especially if a patient is shown appropriate exercises they can carry out. Physiotherapy is likely to be beneficial for patients already experiencing problems with gait and balance, and those who are finding it difficult to initiate movement.

Speech and language therapy

Speech and language therapists can have a crucial role to play in patients whose Parkinson's disease severely affects their speech and ability to communicate effectively. Parkinson's disease often affects control of speech musculature resulting in dysarthria. Amongst other things, speech becomes slurred and monotonal and lacks good articulation making it difficult to be understood. Teaching patients how to project the voice as well as speaking more clearly and slowly can greatly facilitate communication. This is achieved by carrying out specific exercises, which includes exercising the lips, tongue and jaw in order to maintain strength in muscles affected by hypokinesia. A form of therapy called Lee Silverman Voice Therapy (LSVT) can substantially improve speech. Strong commitment is required on the part of the patient since the course is hard work and it is necessary to attend sessions four times a week for several weeks. Unfortunately, this form of treatment is not yet widely available in the UK. Speech and language therapists are able to advise on many techniques that patients can use. Many are straightforward such as swallowing any saliva in the mouth and taking a breath before starting to speak; using short phrases and sentences; and inflecting the voice as much as possible. In cases where speech problems are very severe, speech and language therapists are able to recommend aids such as voice amplifiers and various other communication devices. Being unable to communicate effectively can cause great frustration and feelings of isolation, which should not be underestimated.

Speech and language therapists can also provide help for patients suffering with dysphagia. Swallowing difficulties are common in Parkinson's disease and are probably associated with a reduction in ability to form a bolus in the mouth for swallowing, as well as decreased oesophageal motility. Coughing and spluttering when eating is embarrassing for patients and can also lead to choking. Pneumonia is a frequent cause of death in patients with Parkinson's disease. It has been suggested that aspiration caused by dysphagia is the cause of this high incidence of pneumonia. Speech and language therapists can teach patients an effective swallowing technique. They can also recommend suitable foods and ways of preparing them in order to make the consistency such that they can be more easily swallowed. Dieticians are also able to advise on this and additionally make recommendations about diet.

Occupational therapy

A patient's self-esteem is significantly enhanced by maintaining their ability to do things for themselves. Except for the most disabled, this includes planning their day and carrying out activities whether it be work, hobbies, leisure or just general looking after themselves. The occupational therapist can be a tremendous help in supporting patients to maximise such activities and maintain a level of self-care despite the symptoms of their Parkinson's disease. Occupational therapists help patients to adapt by learning new skills in order to carry out daily activities. If necessary, occupational therapists can organise the supply of special equipment enabling patients to maintain their independence. Aids such as reaching-tongs and devices to help dressing are examples of simple equipment which can dramatically increase the chance of beating the obstacles created by reduced mobility and decreased control of movement. If a patient's disease is progressing significantly, it is important that regular reviews are carried out to ensure any new measures that become necessary are implemented. This is important not only for optimising patient independence, but also for identifying any new risks that may compromise safety.

Complementary and alternative therapies

It has been estimated that 40% of patients who have Parkinson's disease try some form of complementary therapy at some stage. The more common forms of complementary and alternative medicine are outlined below.

Chiropractic

Chiropractic treatment can be useful in alleviating musculoskeletal problems such as back pain. The technique involves gently manipulating the spine to make specific adjustments. Often these help 'free up' any pressure there may be on nerves, which can cause various neurological symptoms including pain. The procedures may not be suitable in patients who have osteoporosis. Although chiropractic treatment can be used on various parts of the body, its main value is in reducing acute pain in the lower back. A survey carried out by the Parkinson's Disease Society in the UK showed that three-quarters of patients with Parkinson's disease considered spinal manipulation to be beneficial.[1]

Osteopathy

Osteopathy is considered by many to be very similar to chiropractic treatment and in as much that they both focus on the misalignment of bones, especially in the spine, they are. However the technique of osteopathy concentrates more on slower, rhythmic stretching and mobilising which subsequently increases the body's ability to regain good health. The osteopathic approach tends to be less 'direct' on specific muscles and joints than with chiropractic treatment. As with chiropractic treatment, osteopathy may not be suitable in patients with osteoporosis.

Alexander technique

The Alexander technique helps improve posture and muscle activity. A controlled trial carried out in patients with Parkinson's disease showed that the Alexander technique was more effective in reducing disability than massage.[2] The Alexander technique may not only have beneficial effects in dealing with the physical aspects of Parkinson's disease, but also help create a more positive approach to dealing with the condition.

Yoga

Yoga focuses on relaxation, breathing and posture and it has been suggested that it may help maintain balance in conditions such as Parkinson's disease. Somewhat surprisingly, a survey carried out by the Parkinson's Disease Society indicated that yoga was considered to be the most effective of the complementary therapies looked at.[1]

Reflexology

There is no good evidence that reflexology is of value in Parkinson's disease. However, some patients consider that it is beneficial and that it helps improve their condition. Reflexology involves massaging areas of the foot in the belief that this affects other parts of the body.

Massage

Therapeutic massage is found by many to be very effective in easing symptoms of muscle pain and stiffness. The patient survey carried out by the Parkinson's Disease Society showed that over 90% of patients gained benefit from massage.[1] See also Aromatherapy below.

Aromatherapy

The main value of aromatherapy probably comes from the pleasant sense of relaxation induced by the smell of the essential oils that are used. If the oils are used during massage, it is understandable that patients believe aromatherapy helps their condition, since massage itself is very effective for reducing muscle stiffness and pain (see above). Aromatherapy can be a very pleasant experience and if nothing else, the feeling of wellbeing and relaxation should not be undervalued.

Acupuncture

There is much controversy concerning the effectiveness of acupuncture for treating Parkinson's disease. Many patients consider it worthless and a waste of money, others feel it provides some benefit for chronic pain. Scientific evidence for this form of therapy is lacking, apart from some data indicating that it can have beneficial effects on sleep.[3] However a double-blind, randomised study comparing acupuncture to a control non-acupuncture procedure, failed to show any statistically significant improvements in the Unified Parkinson's Disease Rating Scale (UPDRS) motor subscale, the Parkinson's Disease Questionnaire (PDQ 39) or the Geriatric Depression Scale.[4] The procedure involves inserting needles at certain points along meridians, the channels through which Chi flows. Chi is considered by traditional Chinese acupuncturists to be the life force which, if disturbed, results in disease. Sticking needles into certain meridians supposedly restores normal flow of Chi.

Homeopathy

Many healthcare professionals and patients consider homeopathic therapies to be little more than placebos and any claimed benefit to be the result of the so-called placebo effect. Scientifically it is difficult to explain how highly diluted compounds can produce a 'pharmacological' action. Despite this, homeopaths and a substantial proportion of patients do believe homeopathic treatments to be efficacious. The muscle cramps suffered by patients with Parkinson's disease is an example of a symptom that some people believe is helped by homeopathic remedies such as *Cuprum*. Some patients use *Argentum nitricum* for treating ataxia and *Causticum* when sleep is disturbed by restless legs.

Herbalism

Unlike homeopathic treatments, herbal remedies can produce unwanted effects and occasionally these can be quite serious. They are usually taken as dried extracts (e.g. powders or capsules) or tinctures. Many herbal preparations are available which are not specifically for the treatment of Parkinson's disease, but for symptoms that occur with numerous conditions. Ginseng for example is widely used by people who feel excessively tired, and *Ginkgo biloba*, which has antioxidant properties, is found by some people to improve mental concentration. A patient with Parkinson's disease suffering with symptoms such as these may consider trying such remedies. Not only can herbal treatments cause adverse effects, but some have the potential to interact with conventional medication. This problem can be illustrated with St John's Wort (*Hypericum perforatum*) which is widely used and has very significant interactions with a large number of drugs including amitriptyline and selective serotonin reuptake inhibitor (SSRI) antidepressants, antiepileptic drugs, 5-hydroxytryptamine $(5\text{-HT})_1$-agonists such as sumatriptan, digoxin, simvastatin and many more. Advice should be sought from a pharmacist before patients take herbal remedies while they are on conventional drug therapy.

See Box 4.1 for a summary of further complementary therapies that may be helpful in patients suffering with Parkinson's disease.

Specific supplements for Parkinson's disease

Although at present there is little scientific evidence that supplements are useful in treating Parkinson's disease,[5] many patients do try them, and some have enormous faith in their benefits. It is important therefore that healthcare professionals who are involved with patients suffering with Parkinson's disease have some knowledge of the preparations in use and an understanding of the basis for their claimed effectiveness. It is conceivable that one day, evidence will become available showing the clinical value of some of these supplements since with many of them there is a degree of theoretical logic for their use.

Box 4.1 Summary of complementary therapies not discussed in the text which may be helpful in patients suffering with Parkinson's disease

Art therapy
An art therapist works with the patient to facilitate self-expression. 'Art in Parkinson's' groups have been established in the UK. Art therapy helps reduce stress and promotes relaxation.

Ayurveda
An ancient Indian healing system. It involves a variety of healing interventions such as changes in lifestyle and diet, the use of herbal remedies (e.g. extracts from the seeds of Mucana plant), exercise and meditation.

Bowen technique
Small gentle movements made to muscles and tendons using the fingers and thumbs. There is anecdotal evidence that it is of value in treating symptoms such as stiffness.

Conductive education
Concentrates on training people how to overcome problems associated with neurological disorders. Sessions especially designed for patients with Parkinson's disease have been established by the National Institute of Conductive Education. There is much anecdotal evidence of benefits to patients with Parkinson's disease.

Feldenkrais method
Similar to the Alexander technique. Focuses on posture, movement and spatial orientation.

Hynotherapy
Useful for symptoms of anxiety and for alleviating both acute and chronic pain. Many patients seem to benefit from hypnotherapy.

Kinesiology
Reflex and acupressure points are used to stimulate natural healing processes. This is combined with body movements and attention to nutrition.

Meditation
Creates a sense of calm which helps symptom of stress. Benefits are physical, psychological and spiritual.

Music therapy
Can help improve mobility, speech and promote relaxation. Music with a strong beat can help patients with Parkinson's disease improve their walking and overcome 'freezing' episodes. Published studies confirm benefit in Parkinson's disease.

continued overleaf

Box 4.1 Continued

Pilates
Improves postures, muscle strength and flexibility. The exercises are carried out on a floor mat or in specialist studios with specialist equipment for applying pressure to joints.

Reiki
A healer places their hands above the patient who 'draws out' energy. There are anecdotal claims that pain due to rigidity is improved.

Shiatsu
Involves holding or pressing on the meridians to improve 'energy flow'. Sometimes involves rotations and stretches. It may aid relaxation, sleeping and posture.

Tai chi
Consists of 'centring' the mind and the body. There is evidence of improvement in walking and sleeping and reduction in falls.

Yoga
An integrated approach of mind and body control. It may be helpful in treating anxiety and depression.

Notes
- This list is not exhaustive and does not include information on all complementary therapies that might be available.
- For more details of complementary therapies, readers are referred to an excellent booklet published by the Parkinson's Disease Society of Great Britain in October 2005 called *Complementary Therapies in Parkinson's Disease*.

Coenzyme Q_{10}

Coenzyme Q_{10} has been used for many years by patients with Parkinson's disease. It is readily available and stocked by most health-food stores. Coenzyme Q_{10} is also known as ubiquinone, a name given to reflect the fact it is ubiquitous in cells of the body where it is involved in the processes of producing energy by mitochondria; coenzyme Q_{10} seems to act as a catalyst to the biochemical steps involved. Some studies have shown that levels of coenzyme Q_{10} are reduced in patients suffering with Parkinson's disease. Other work suggests that mitochondrial function is impaired in Parkinson's disease. Clearly these two discoveries could well be linked. Furthermore, reduced activity within mitochondria can lead to excessive concentrations of free radicals, which are known to cause cell damage. It is conceivable this plays a part in the progression of the disease, by causing degeneration of the neuronal pathways involved in the control of movement. This provides the rationale for patients using coenzyme Q_{10} in an attempt to reduce disease progression.

The coenzyme Q_{10} preparations available in health-food stores are usually in 30 mg or 60 mg strengths. The scientific evidence suggesting that coenzyme Q_{10} may slow the progression of Parkinson's disease, was generated in studies using much larger doses up to 1.2 g daily, and even then the results were not conclusive. Whether the low-strength preparations commercially available have any useful effect is doubtful. Coenzyme Q_{10} is present in a number of foods including beef, sardines, mackerel and peanuts, but in even smaller amounts, so the likelihood of a diet modified to increase the dietary intake of coenzyme Q_{10} being effective in Parkinson's disease is remote.

The first study showing evidence that coenzyme Q_{10} could slow the decline of progression of Parkinson's disease was published in 2002.[6] Three dose levels were used, 300 mg, 600 mg and 1.2 g daily. Patients receiving the lower two doses had an outcome no different from those on placebo. However, patients receiving 1.2 g daily had a significantly lower score on the UPDRS than the others, which was concluded to mean the disease had progressed less. Motor symptoms, mental well-being and ability to perform activities were all significantly different in patients taking the higher dose. Many regard the results from this study as encouraging, but clearly more data need to be generated to confirm the beneficial effects of coenzyme Q_{10}. Side-effects were minimal, and problems with indigestion were usually solved by taking the preparation with meals.

Vitamin E

As with many vitamins and other supplements, vitamin E has been the subject of substantial research, much of it focusing on its antioxidant properties. The well known DATATOP study (Deprenyl and Tocopherol Antioxidative Therapy of Parkinsonism) examined the effect of selegiline (deprenyl) and tocopherol on disease progression.[7] Tocopherol is one of the more important and biologically active forms of vitamin E. It was concluded from this large study involving 800 patients that tocopherol had no useful effect in delaying the progression of Parkinson's disease. Furthermore, suggestions that selegiline was shown to produce a neuroprotective effect are widely disputed. Later-published work has further confirmed that tocopherol is ineffective in slowing the degenerative processes occurring in Parkinson's disease.[8] Advocates of vitamin E claim that the reason no benefit was found in these studies is that synthetic tocopherol was used rather than vitamin E in its natural form. More recent studies of patients eating foods high in vitamin E have produced interesting results,[9] but whether any observed influence on the disease was due to the higher vitamin E intake is unclear.

A systematic review and meta-analysis of observational studies suggests that vitamin E does offer protection against Parkinson's disease.[10] The authors concluded that this may be the result of neuro-protective effects reducing the risks of Parkinson's disease developing, but admit that randomised controlled trials would be needed to confirm this suggestion.

In misguided enthusiasm for this form of treatment, some patients have taken high doses of vitamin E which have been sufficient to result in adverse effects. Gastrointestinal upset and abdominal pain can occur and some patients have experienced blurred vision, dizziness and weakness.

Glutathione

When administered by injection, there is some evidence that glutathione helps a number of conditions. However, when taken orally as a supplement, confirmation of useful therapeutic effect is lacking. This is probably due to it being broken down in the gastrointestinal tract. Supplements of N-acetylcysteine increase the production of glutathione in the body, but again there is little evidence for significant benefits on the symptoms of Parkinson's disease.

S-adenosylmethionine (SAMe)

During the search for new ways of increasing antioxidant intake with a view to delaying the progression of Parkinson's disease, S-adenosyl-methionine (often abbreviated to SAMe – pronounced as 'Sammy') was found to reduce oxidative stress in laboratory animals. Subsequently, some patients use SAMe as a dietary supplement, but the usefulness of this is far from certain. The only research into its potential effects on motor function in Parkinson's disease has been carried out in the laboratory, and the results from this work are not encouraging. It has been tried in humans to see if it improved the depression that can be associated with Parkinson's disease.[11] However, the trial was so small and badly designed, that the positive results obtained are not considered to be helpful in supporting the use of this compound.

Green tea

Green tea comes from the tea plant *Camellia sinensis*. The leaves are allowed to wither and then steamed, not fermented like the leaves used to produce black tea. Tea derived from *Camellia sinensis* contains high levels of polyphenols. Polyphenols are powerful antioxidants and in the body act as free-radical scavengers preventing damage occurring to cells. It may not be a coincidence that the prevalence of Parkinson's disease is much lower in Asia and Africa where green tea is commonly drunk.

Fermented papaya

Some years back, publicity was given to the use of fermented papaya extract by Pope John Paul II who allegedly took it to relieve symptoms of his Parkinson's disease. It was prescribed as a 'miracle treatment' by a French doctor during an audience with the Pope to discuss the problem of AIDS in Africa. It was claimed the product possessed antioxidant properties, hence the rationale for its use. Such publicity not only inappropriately raised the hopes of people with the disease that the preparation is effective, but has led to misunderstanding and confusion about its availability in health-food shops. The so-called papaya enzyme products are not the same as the fermented papaya extract which it is thought the Pope used.

References

1. Brown R. The role of complementary therapy in Parkinson's disease. *Geriatr Med* 1998; 28: 63–67.
2. Stallibrass C, Sissons P, Chalmers C. Randomised controlled trial of the Alexander technique for idiopathic Parkinson's disease. *Clin Rehabil* 2002; 16: 695–708.
3. Shulman LM, Wen X, Weiner WJ, *et al*. Acupuncture therapy for the symptoms of Parkinson's disease. *Mov Disord* 2002; 17: 799–802.
4. Cristian A, Katz M, Cutrone E, Walker RH. Evaluation of acupuncture in the treatment of Parkinson's disease: a double-blind pilot study. *Mov Disord* 2005; 20: 1185–1188.
5. Suchowersky O, Gronseth G, Perlmutter J, *et al*. Practice parameter: neuro-protective strategies and alternative therapies for Parkinson disease (an evidence-based review): report of the Quality Standards Subcommittee of the American Academy of Neurology. *Neurology* 2006; 66: 976–982.

6.   Shults CW, Oakes D, Kieburtz K, *et al.* Effects of coenzyme Q10 in early Parkinson's disease: evidence of slowing of the functional decline. *Arch Neurol* 2002; 59:1541–1550.

7.   The Parkinson Study Group. Effect of deprenyl on the progression of disability in early Parkinson's disease. *N Engl J Med* 1989; 321: 1364–1371.

8.   The Parkinson Study Group. Effects of tocopherol and deprenyl on the progression of disability in early Parkinson's disease. *N Engl J Med* 1993; 328: 176–183.

9.   Zhang SM, Hernan MA, Chen H, *et al.* Intakes of vitamins E and C, carotenoids, vitamin supplements and PD risk. *Neurology* 2002; 59: 1161–1169.

10.   Etminan M, Gill S, Samii A. Intake of vitamin E, vitamin C, and carotenoids and the risk of Parkinson's disease: a meta-analysis. *Lancet Neurol* 2005; 4: 362–365.

11.   Di Rocco A, Rogers JD, Brown R, *et al.* S-adenosyl-methionine improves depression in patients with Parkinson's disease in an open-label clinical trial. *Mov Disord* 2000; 15: 1225–1229.

Further reading

Deane HO, Ellis-Hill C, Dekker K, *et al.* A survey of current OT practice for Parkinson's Disease in the UK. *Br J Occup Ther* 2003; 66: 193–200.

Ramig LO, Sapir S, Countryman S, *et al.* Intensive voice treatment (LSVT) for patients with Parkinson's disease: a 2 year follow up. *J Neurol Neurosurg Psychiatry* 2001; 71: 493–498.

5

Surgical procedures

Attempts to alleviate the symptoms of Parkinson's disease with surgery date back to the 1940s. This was 20 years or so prior to the introduction of therapy with levodopa, so an effective treatment was anxiously sought. However, the beneficial effects of these early surgical procedures were negligible and were associated with a high rate of mortality and substantial morbidity. The techniques that were employed consisted primarily of lesioning areas of the brain (the motor cortex and the dendate nucleus of the cerebellum) and pathways in the spinal cord. In the 1950s, slightly more successful attempts were made by making lesions in the globus pallidus. The discovery in the 1960s that levodopa was a successful treatment for Parkinson's disease diverted interest towards drug therapy, and less attention was paid to developing surgical techniques. For many years, any work carried out on surgical measures was essentially overshadowed by the enthusiasm to optimise the use of levodopa and find other drugs that might have a useful effect on the disease. However, interest in surgery become renewed when it was realised that levodopa, and other drugs subsequently introduced, had limitations and did not provide the answer for patients severely affected by Parkinson's disease. Advances in stereotactic surgery also provided the motivation to experiment further with surgical techniques. Stereotaxis is a method which enables very precise three-dimensional targeting of, for example, a probe used to lesion a certain area of the brain. Complex computerised imaging using computerised tomography (CT) or magnetic resonance imaging (MRI) scans provide the necessary 'map'. The more accurate targeting using stereotaxis increased the likelihood of a successful outcome and reduced the risk of affecting other areas of the brain with potentially disastrous consequences.

Referral to the diagram shown on Plate 9 will help identify those areas of the brain primarily involved in the pathophysiology of Parkinson's disease (see Chapter 2 for more details). The primary loop in the brain responsible for controlling movement runs from the premotor cortex to the striatum, then on to the globus pallidus and from there to the thalamus, which in turn feeds back to the motor cortex. Activity in this loop is influenced by one mechanism acting as an accelerator (the substantia nigra), and another acting like a brake (the subthalamic nucleus). In Parkinson's disease, degeneration of the nigrostriatal pathway effectively means the accelerator to the loop is not functioning. This situation can be counteracted and some balance regained in the loop, by reducing the activity of the pathway from the subthalamic nucleus to the globus pallidus (i.e. reducing the braking mechanism). Alternatively, activity in the part of the loop running from the globus pallidus to the thalamus could be reduced, producing a similar effect. In Parkinson's disease there are therefore three areas of overactivity in the brain which result in inappropriate activity from the thalamus to the motor cortex slowing the patient down and producing the characteristic symptoms of the disease:

- the subthalamic nucleus
- the globus pallidus
- the thalamus.

These three sites therefore form the targets for surgical inactivation. There are two ways in which this inactivation can be achieved. Firstly by lesioning which is achieved by inserting a probe through a burr hole in the skull to one of the sites cited above, and passing an electrical current though the tip which then heats up and destroys the tissue in contact with the end of the probe. In line with the three areas of the brain listed above, this procedure is known as:

- subthalamotomy
- pallidotomy
- thalamotomy.

Another technique is to place a permanent electrode in one of the above areas of the brain and connect this to an electrical stimulator similar to a pacemaker. High-frequency electrical impulses are delivered to the electrode in order to overstimulate the site where the tip is. This causes a depolarising block and thereby reduces conduction in the pathway. In line with the three areas of the brain listed above, this procedure is known as:

- subthalamic stimulation
- pallidal stimulation
- thalamic stimulation.

The general term used to describe this technique is deep brain stimulation (DBS) and, unlike lesioning, it is reversible since the tissue is not destroyed. For this reason and the fact that stimulation of the areas of the brain is associated with a lower morbidity, DBS has become the preferred method.

The risks

Although surgical techniques are much more advanced now, there is obviously a degree of risk associated with the procedures outlined above. All of them are therefore reserved for patients with severely disabling symptoms. Bleeding into an area of the brain, causing a stroke, is a significant risk and occurs in 2–3% of patients. However, mortality from these surgical procedures is now less than 1%. Patients who undergo a bilateral procedure (both sides of the brain being targeted) have a higher risk of complications. For example, less than 10% of patients who have a unilateral procedure experience difficulties afterwards with swallowing and find their speech is affected. However, the likelihood of such problems increases to up to 30% in patients who have a bilateral procedure. Similarly, adverse effects on memory are more severe in patients who have received treatment on both sides of the brain. Some of the unwanted effects following surgery, such as confusion, seizures and facial weakness, are often transient.

Ablative surgery

Subthalamotomy

At the present time, there is little experience in humans of directly targeting the subthalamic nucleus and performing a subthalamotomy. Subthalamotomy carried out in animal models of Parkinson's disease (induced with 1-methyl-4-phenyl-1,2,3,6-tetrahydropyridine (MPTP)) have been successful. However, there are fears that lesioning the subthalamic nucleus may cause a hemiballismus/hemichorea syndrome. This syndrome occurs in patients who have suffered a stroke in this area of the brain, hence the procedure is carried out in only a few centres where the benefits and risks are being assessed.

Pallidotomy

Unlike subthalamotomy, there is much more experience in carrying out pallidotomy, and substantially more evidence is available regarding the value and the complications of the operation. The procedure normally carried out is a posteroventral pallidotomy (PVP), a term which describes the location in the globus pallidus interna where the lesion is made. It is usually an effective treatment, and four out of every five patients obtain substantial improvement in the dyskinesia resulting from levodopa therapy. Furthermore, the beneficial effects are long-lasting. Improvement in symptoms is most noticeable on the opposite side of the body (contralateral) to where the lesion is made. Improvements on the same side (ipsilateral) are transient and less dramatic. Other symptoms that may improve a little include rigidity, bradykinesia and tremor. Again, any improvement is usually short-lived. Patients who experience pain from muscle spasm and rigidity often find this is greatly reduced following pallidotomy. Symptoms that occur during the 'off' phase, such as freezing, are helped bilaterally, often improving the patient's ability to perform activities of daily living. However, the major benefit is a reduction in dyskinesia during the 'on' phase. For some patients this means that the dosage of levodopa can be increased since they are able to take larger amounts before the problems of dyskinesia limit further increases.

Pallidotomy carries a risk of causing visual field defects and hemi-paresis, and as with similar surgery to other parts of the brain, there is a risk of intracerebral haemorrhage. Mortality from the procedure is around 2% and the chance of serious disability occurring is approxi-mately 5%.

It is rare for the operation to be performed bilaterally as this substantially increases the risk of swallowing (dysphagia) and speaking difficulties (dysphonia).

Thalamotomy

The area of the thalamus which is targeted for lesioning is the ventro-intermediate nucleus (VIM). This results in a dramatic decrease of tremor, sometimes to the point of eliminating it altogether. The success of this treatment is usually maintained for a long time; however, in a small proportion of patients the tremor returns after only a few months. The lesion is made on the opposite side (contralateral) of the brain to the side of the body most affected by tremor. Bilateral surgery is some-times performed in cases of severe tremor affecting both sides of the body. However, the development of dysarthria (slurred speech) is more common following bilateral thalamotomy. Symptoms of rigidity, hypo-kinesia and bradykinesia are not significantly helped by thalamotomy.

Deep brain stimulation

Instead of destroying an area of tissue within the brain as outlined previously (pallidotomy, thalamotomy, subthalamotomy), an electrical current can be applied to the targeted area. By varying the nature and amplitude of the pulses, a depolarising block is established in the pathway at the site where the electrical stimulation is applied. In practice this is achieved by inserting a probe into the brain so that the tip enters the appropriate area. This is left *in situ* and connected to a pulse generator (stimulator) which is implanted under the skin (see Plates 10, 11 and 13). The nature of the electrical current is programmed after the surgery to obtain maximum clinical benefit for the patient. The battery in the implant device delivering the electrical current usually lasts between 3 and 5 years. Complications arising from implanting the probe and stimulator device are rare; however, if these become infected, their removal becomes necessary.

Thalamic stimulation

The target for thalamic stimulation is the same as that for thalamotomy – the VIM. As with thalamotomy, substantial improvement of tremor is achieved in most patients. Some improvement may be seen in dyskinesia, but other symptoms of Parkinson's disease are rarely improved. The risks associated with inserting the electrode are the same as with thalamotomy. Intracerebral bleeds occur in about 2% of cases and speech, swallowing and memory may be affected. During the programming phase after surgery, the patient often experiences tingling and numbness; sometimes adverse effects affecting vision occur. Adverse events related to stimulation were significantly more frequent in patients stimulated bilaterally compared to those undergoing unilateral stimulation.[1] The guideline published in 2006 for the diagnosis and management of Parkinson's disease in primary and secondary care recommended that thalamic stimulation be considered in patients with severe disabling tremor when it is not possible to perform stimulation of the subthalamic nucleus.[2]

Pallidal stimulation

The beneficial effects of pallidal stimulation are similar to those of pallidotomy. Levodopa-induced dyskinesia is effectively reduced. However, there is much variation in how successfully other symptoms associated with Parkinson's disease are controlled. Optimising the settings of the stimulator can be difficult, maximal control of dyskinesia often being compromised by a worsening in bradykinesia. At present this procedure is rarely carried out in the UK, but it may be a suitable alternative to stimulation of the subthalamic nucleus when this is not possible.

Subthalamic stimulation

The technique of stimulating the subthalamic nucleus is developing, though experience is somewhat limited at present. A study of 100 patients showed significant clinical improvement with reduction in dyskinesias, and the duration and severity of 'off' state.[3] The main problems encountered were device infections and hardware problems such as battery failure. A 5-year follow-up study in patients who were treated with stimulation of the subthalamic nucleus suggests that improvement in motor function is maintained for at least 5 years.[4] A study comparing the outcomes from pallidal stimulation (stimulation of the globus pallidus interna) and stimulation of the subthalamic nucleus showed that bradykinesia was improved more by the latter.[5] However, more comparative studies are needed before it can be concluded that subthalamic nucleus stimulation is superior. In 2003 the National Institute for Clinical Excellence (NICE) published a statement on bilateral stimulation of the subthalamic nucleus supporting the use of this procedure providing all the appropriate safeguards and processes for audit are in place.[6]

The PD SURG trial[7] recruited patients up until 2006. Hopefully, when the results are available (expected 2008), they will provide valuable information on the clinical outcomes and health-economic aspects. The guideline published in 2006 for the diagnosis and management of Parkinson's disease in primary and secondary care suggests that bilateral stimulation of the subthalamic nucleus may be suitable for patients who have motor complications not responding to optimised drug treatment, and are responsive to levodopa.[8] Its use in patients with depression, dementia or other mental health problems is not recommended.

References

1.	Krauss JK, Simpson RK Jr, Ondo WG, *et al.* Concepts and methods in chronic thalamic stimulation for treatment of tremor: technique and application. *Neurosurgery* 2001; 48: 535–541.

2. National Collaborating Centre for Chronic Conditions. *Parkinson's Disease: diagnosis and management in primary and secondary care* [full guideline]. London: National Collaborating Centre for Chronic Conditions, 2006, 111.
3. Goodman RR, Kim B, McClelland S, *et al*. Operative techniques and morbidity with subthalamic nucleus deep brain stimulation in 100 consecutive patients with advanced Parkinson's disease. *J Neurol Neurosurg Psychiatry* 2006; 77: 12–17.
4. Schupbach WM, Chastan N, Welter ML, *et al*. Stimulation of the subthalamic nucleus in Parkinson's disease: a 5 year follow up. *J Neurol Neurosurg Psychiatry* 2005; 76: 1640–1644.
5. Anderson VC, Burchiel KJ, Hogarth P, *et al*. Pallidal vs subthalamic nucleus deep brain stimulation in Parkinson disease. *Arch Neurol* 2005; 62: 554–560.
6. National Institute of Clinical Excellence. *Deep Brain Stimulation for Parkinson's Disease* (IPG 019). London: NICE, 2003.
7. www.pdsurg.bham.ac.uk/ (accessed 7 June 2007).
8. National Collaborating Centre for Chronic Conditions. *Parkinson's Disease: diagnosis and management in primary and secondary care* [full guideline]. London: National Collaborating Centre for Chronic Conditions, 2006, 107.

Further reading

Alvarez L, Macias R, Lopez G, *et al*. Bilateral subthalamotomy in Parkinson's disease: initial and long-term response. *Brain* 2005; 128: 570–583.

Colnat-Coulbois S, Gauchard GC, Maillard L, *et al*. Bilateral subthalamic nucleus stimulation improves balance control in Parkinson's disease. *J Neurol Neurosurg Psychiatry* 2005; 76: 780–787.

Diamond A, Jankovic J. The effect of deep brain stimulation on quality of life in movement disorders. *J Neurol Neurosurg Psychiatry* 2005; 76:1188–1193.

Ohye C, Shibazaki T, Sato S. Gamma knife thalamotomy for movement disorders: evaluation of the thalamic lesion and clinical results. *J Neurosurg* 2005; 102 (Suppl): 234–240.

Rodriguez-Oroz MC, Obeso JA, Lang AE, *et al*. Bilateral deep brain stimulation in Parkinson's disease: a multicentre study with 4 years follow-up. *Brain* 2005; 128: 2240–2249.

Walter BL, Vitek JL. Surgical treatment for Parkinson's disease. *Lancet Neurol* 2004; 3: 719–728.

6

Management of non-motor symptoms

In addition to the motor symptoms characteristic of patients with Parkinson's disease, other symptoms often emerge. These usually develop as the disease progresses, but sometimes occur in the earlier stages. It is not unusual for the non-motor symptoms to actually be more troublesome in advanced Parkinson's disease than the motor symptoms. They are often the cause of significant reductions in quality of life, add substantially to disability and may reduce life expectancy.[1] The impact of these symptoms may be underestimated if the prime focus of attention is on the effects Parkinson's disease has on motor function. This can be unfortunate for the patient, since therapy for many of the non-motor symptoms can be very successful and greatly improve the patient's wellbeing.

Neuropsychiatric manifestations of Parkinson's disease include depression, sleep disorders, psychosis, anxiety disorders, dementia and sexual disorders.[2] Although tools exist to screen for depression, psychosis and dementia, in patients with Parkinson's disease more specific validated methods are needed.[3] Many of the drugs used to treat Parkinson's disease can themselves precipitate hallucinations, paranoid delusions and mania. The development of severe psychosis is often the condition which makes it necessary for a patient with Parkinson's disease to be cared for in a nursing home. Unfortunately, such a move often leads to further confusion for the patient due to unfamiliar surroundings.

This chapter reviews the more common non-motor symptoms of Parkinson's disease and their management.

Constipation

The presence of Lewy bodies in parts of the gastrointestinal tract supports the belief that Parkinson's disease can directly affect the nerves controlling gastrointestinal function. Patients with Parkinson's disease often suffer with constipation that is severe enough to warrant remedial steps. Rather surprisingly, constipation can become a substantial problem in the early stages of the disease. In many cases, increasing fluid and fibre intake will be sufficient to resolve the problem and these measures should always be tried first. Only if these steps prove to be inadequate, should a laxative be taken. Providing a patient achieves at least three bowel movements each week by maintaining healthy and regular eating habits, a high-fibre diet and a reasonable degree of exercise, laxatives are best reserved for any episodes of more severe constipation. If regular laxative use is necessary, this does not mean that the more natural methods can be abandoned; they should still be used in order that the dosage of laxative needed can be kept to a minimum. In severe cases of constipation, more than one laxative may be needed, in which case drugs with different modes of action should be used. Details of the most commonly used laxatives are given below.

Bulk-forming laxatives

These agents improve peristalsis by increasing faecal mass. Several days may elapse before maximum effect is obtained. This form of laxative is particularly suitable for patients who produce small hard stools. Ideally the increase in bulk should be achieved by including sufficient fibre in the diet, rather than taking medication. It is important that adequate fluid intake is maintained otherwise intestinal obstruction can occur following the use of bulk-forming laxatives.

Preparations of ispaghula husk, sterculia and methylcellulose are available. The first two agents are normally taken as granules or powder mixed with water; methylcellulose is taken in tablet form with at least 300 ml of water.

Stimulant laxatives

Of the anthraquinone group, only senna is widely used, dantron being reserved for use in constipation of terminally ill patients due to concerns about its carcinogenic properties. Senna usually acts within 8–12 h. Bisacodyl can be taken orally, in which case it acts within 10–12 h. When administered as a suppository it can produce the desired effect in as little as 20 min and rarely takes longer than 1 h. Glycerol suppositories work by producing a mild irritant effect in the rectum. In addition to a stimulant action, docusate sodium also works as a softening agent. It can take 1 or 2 days before docusate sodium has a useful effect.

Since these agents increase intestinal motility, it is not uncommon for them to cause abdominal cramps. In some patients, continual use can lead to diarrhoea and hypokalaemia.

Faecal softeners

As mentioned above, docusate sodium softens stools as well as having an effect as a stimulant laxative. Arachis oil enemas are reserved for softening impacted faeces. Liquid paraffin is not recommended for long-term use since it can cause anal irritation and affects the absorption of fat-soluble vitamins. Lipoid pneumonia and granulomatous reaction have been reported.

Osmotic laxatives

Lactulose takes up to 2 days to produce its effect. This, together with its potential side-effects including abdominal cramps and flatulence, limits the use of lactulose and it is not recommended as a first-choice preparation. Macrogol preparations are useful for chronic constipation and are taken in the form of a powder mixed with water. Abdominal discomfort and nausea may limit their use.

Sialorrhoea

Up to 80% of patients have problems with excessive saliva and drooling. For some reason it occurs more commonly in men. In addition to help from speech and language therapists in increasing swallowing, sub-lingual atropine solution (e.g. using 1% eye drops) twice daily may be effective.[4]

Urinary problems

Detrusor hyper-reflexia may occur as a problem associated with Parkinson's disease. It is likely that the cause for this originates from changes occurring in the area of the micturition centre in the brain. If severe urinary symptoms occur at the early stages of Parkinson's disease, other causes such as prostate problems should be excluded; a diagnosis of multiple system atrophy (MSA) should also be considered.

Patients experience urgency and urge incontinence, often with frequency and nocturia. Drug therapy is effective in many, but not all, patients. Furthermore, side-effects can be troublesome.

Oxybutynin increases bladder capacity and also decreases the effect of detrusor hyper-reflexia. An oral dose of 2.5–5 mg twice or three times daily may be sufficient, though a dosage of up to 5 mg four times daily can be taken. A modified-release preparation is available and is claimed to produce fewer side-effects. The dosage as modified-release tablets is 5 mg daily increased if necessary at weekly intervals up to a maximum of 20 mg daily. More recently, a transdermal patch has been marketed. A new patch is applied twice a week to dry unbroken skin on the abdomen, hip or buttock. Each patch contains 36 mg of oxybutynin which is released at a rate of 3.9 mg over 24 h. The site of application should be rotated, the same site being avoided for at least 7 days.

Tolterodine has similar effects to oxybutynin, but may be better tolerated in some patients. Normally the dosage is 2 mg twice daily, though this should be reduced to 1 mg twice daily if side-effects are troublesome at the higher dose. A modified-release preparation of tolterodine is available, the dosage of which is 4 mg daily.

Both oxybutynin and tolterodine produce antimuscarinic side-effects including dry mouth, constipation, blurred vision and difficulty in micturition. Since constipation is a very common problem in patients with Parkinson's disease, care should be taken to ensure that any success in reducing urinary problems is not more than offset by more severe problems with constipation. Since antimuscarinic drugs reduce sweating, fainting can occur in hot weather.

Flavoxate is better tolerated, but unfortunately is often ineffective. Other antimuscarinic drugs available include propiverine, solifenacin and trospium.

Depression

The importance of managing depression in patients with Parkinson's disease should not be underestimated. Some studies have shown that the incidence is very high (up to 50%) in these patients.[5] Furthermore, there is good evidence that depression can be a much more significant factor in reducing the quality of life than the motor symptoms associated with Parkinson's disease. It is perhaps understandable that the focus of attention in a neurology clinic is on movement and physical functionality. In attempting to optimise the choice and dosage of anti-Parkinson's drugs, the need for identifying and treating other symptoms can be overshadowed. It is important to look at the whole package of symptoms, especially as many, such as depression, may be improved with appropriate therapy.

It is attractive to believe that the high incidence of depression in patients with Parkinson's disease is a result of decreased activity in dopaminergic pathways. The fact that the antihypertensive drug methyldopa (a false transmitter) frequently causes depression as a side-effect supports this, as does the fact that reserpine which depletes dopamine in the brain is a powerful inducer of depression. However, such a straightforward explanation is unlikely. After all, levodopa therapy itself rarely helps in alleviating the symptoms of depression. The explanation will be much more complex and probably involve other neurotransmitters such as 5-hydroxytryptamine (serotonin) and noradrenaline (epinephrine).

Other causes of depression should be considered. The incidence of hypothyroidism is higher in patients with Parkinson's disease. Since this can result in symptoms of depression, thyroid function should be assessed in patients to rule out this treatable cause. Worry, anxiety and stress are frequent and understandable conditions in patients with Parkinson's disease. Non-drug forms of therapy can have dramatic effects. Reassurance regarding the future, help in planning, and talking through worries and concerns may be the most effective medicine.

There are reports that some symptoms of Parkinson's disease may worsen as a result of antidepressant therapy, particularly with the use of selective serotonin reuptake inhibitors (SSRIs).[6] In view of this, patients should be assessed after commencing antidepressant therapy to ensure, on balance, that the therapy is helpful. The SSRI group includes citalopram, fluoxetine, fluvoxamine, paroxetine and sertraline. These drugs have fewer antimuscarinic side-effects than the tricyclic antidepressants and are less cardiotoxic. The tricyclic antidepressants may be more suitable in patients who have difficulty sleeping since this group of antidepressants tends to have a more sedative effect. However, care should be taken in patients prone to suffer with orthostatic hypotension since tricyclic antidepressants may exacerbate the problem. The tricyclic antidepressants most commonly used are amitriptyline and dosulepin.

The evidence from clinical trials showing the value of antidepressants in patients with Parkinson's disease is very limited. A meta-analysis of trials that have been published showed that placebo and antidepressants were equally effective in treating the depression associated with Parkinson's disease.[7] When used to treat elderly depressed patients who did *not* have Parkinson's disease, those who received active drug gained much more benefit than those receiving placebo. Interestingly, in the group of depressed patients that did have Parkinson's disease, those who gained most benefit were in the older age groups and those who had more severe depression. The study also showed that the newer anti-depressants are well tolerated in Parkinson's disease.

Psychosis

A patient with Parkinson's disease may develop psychosis as a symptom of their disease and/or as an adverse effect to their medication. Psychosis associated with Lewy body dementia is not an uncommon problem occurring with advanced Parkinson's disease. This may not be amenable to treatment, and in some cases the only practical option is provision of an appropriate level of ongoing care, often in a nursing home. However, if medication has been changed in recent weeks, the possibility that this is responsible, or contributing to the problem, should be considered.

Many drugs used to treat Parkinson's disease have the potential to cause symptoms of psychosis. In patients who are younger or only in the early stages of the disease, medication is more likely to be the culprit and should be reviewed. When making changes to a patient's drug therapy for Parkinson's disease, a balance may have to be made between the severity of psychotic symptoms, especially their impact on the patient, and the degree of control achieved in movement symptoms associated with Parkinson's disease.

Unfortunately many of the antipsychotic drugs that might effectively treat psychosis cause a worsening of Parkinson's disease symptoms. Drugs such as the butyrophenones (e.g. haloperidol) increase movement problems, probably by pharmacologically blocking dopamine receptors. Some newer antipsychotic agents, often called 'atypical' antipsychotics, are less of a problem in this respect and are regarded as the treatment of choice.[8]

Quetiapine is often chosen since it is better tolerated than some of the other drugs. The dosage is low at the start of treatment, e.g. 12.5–25 mg daily, but this can be increased to a maintenance dose normally in the range of 50–300 mg daily in two divided doses. Occasionally, doses of up to 400 mg daily in two divided doses are necessary.

Clozapine is also used in these patients, but can cause serious side-effects such as neutropenia and potentially fatal agranulocytosis. Rigorous blood testing is necessary to detect agranulocytosis. For the first 18 weeks of treatment with clozapine, leucocyte and differential blood counts must be done every week. After 18 weeks, the frequency may be reduced to every 2 weeks, and after 1 year blood tests must be performed at least once every 4 weeks. Dosage is started low at 12.5 mg once daily, but this is increased gradually to a dose usually in the range of 25–37.5 mg. Doses as high as 100 mg daily can be used in severe cases following cautious dose increases of 12.5 mg per week.

Drugs such as risperidone and olanzapine are sometimes used but seem to cause deterioration in motor function for a number of patients.

Other triggers of psychotic symptoms should always be ruled out. In the elderly, severe infection or dehydration may be the real cause of psychotic symptoms.

Dementia

Around one in five patients with Parkinson's disease develops dementia in the advanced stages of the disease. Often, these patients are also exhibiting signs of psychosis. Lewy body dementia can produce symptoms such as hallucinations. Since a number of drugs used to treat Parkinson's disease can also precipitate such effects, medication should always be considered as a possible cause and adjusted if appropriate. Often the dementia associated with Parkinson's disease does not follow a steadily progressive course, but is more fluctuating in nature, and compared to Alzheimer's disease, short-term memory is not usually so badly affected.

Drugs marketed for treating Alzheimer's disease have been used to treat Lewy body dementia in Parkinson's disease; however, the true value of these drugs for this indication has yet to be determined. Most of the drugs used to treat Alzheimer's disease inhibit acetylcholinesterase, thereby increasing levels of acetylcholine. In theory, this could potentially worsen the motor symptoms of Parkinson's disease, but little information is available indicating whether this occurs in practice. The main value of drugs used to treat dementia is in enhancing cognition, or at least slowing down progression of this symptom. The true value of these drugs in treating Alzheimer's disease is currently under review and there is very little evidence available supporting their use in dementia associated with Parkinson's disease.

A recent Cochrane review of the published literature found just one randomised, double-blind, placebo-controlled study carried out specifically in patients with Parkinson's disease.[9] This looked at the efficacy of rivastigmine, its safety and tolerability in 541 patients.[10] Rivastigmine produced clinically significant improvements in cognition and activities of daily living in approximately 15% of patients. This improvement in outcome is similar to that seen when rivastigmine is used to treat Alzheimer's disease. However, the drug was poorly tolerated by a large number of patients, nausea, vomiting and tremor being major problems.

These effects were the cause of many patients who had rivastigmine dropping out of the trial.

Since the Cochrane review of the literature was carried out, a further paper has been published assessing the value of donepezil in treating dementia associated with Parkinson's disease.[11] The results of this randomised, double-blind, placebo-controlled, crossover study were not impressive. Only one of the cognitive scales used in the trial showed a statistically significant difference between donepezil and placebo. The drug was well tolerated and did not appear to worsen the motor symptoms of Parkinson's disease. Galantamine produced modest benefits in cognitive outcomes in a study of patients suffering with dementia associated with Parkinson's disease.[12] However, worsening tremor, vomiting and anorexia attributed to the drug resulted in it being discontinued in a number of patients.

Donepezil, galantamine and rivastigmine are all reversible inhibitors of acetylcholinesterase licensed for treating Alzheimer's disease. Galantamine also stimulates nicotinic receptors, but the significance of this in producing useful therapeutic effect is unknown. Memantine is also used to treat Alzheimer's disease, but has a different pharmacological action; it affects transmission in glutamatergic pathways by blocking N-methyl-D-aspartate (NMDA) receptors. It should be noted that all of these drugs are specifically licensed for use in Alzheimer's disease, rather than dementia in general.

Hypotension

Hypotension, particularly orthostatic hypotension, can be a troublesome symptom, especially in patients with severe Parkinson's disease. Drug treatment for motor symptoms of Parkinson's disease can also exacerbate or cause low blood pressure. Other drugs such as tricyclic antidepressants, drugs for cardiac conditions, and diuretics are also potential culprits. Typically, a patient feels faint when rising from a sitting or lying position. In severe cases, a patient may lose consciousness leading to a fall and a high chance of injury. Hot weather and various other factors can increase the likelihood and severity of hypotension. Other medical conditions such as anaemia should also be considered.

All medication being taken by the patient should be reviewed and dosages or choice of drug changed where appropriate. There are also a number of things the patient can do to reduce the problem. Rising slowly when getting up, avoiding hot showers or baths, maintaining adequate hydration, avoiding large meals and being careful with alcohol intake can all help. If troublesome hypotension persists despite the steps outlined above, treatment with fludrocortisone or midodrine may be considered.

The salt-retaining steroid fludrocortisone is effective in some, but not all, patients. By increasing sodium retention, plasma volume is maintained. The dosage is usually between 0.05 mg and 0.2 mg daily. Postural hypotension caused by levodopa might be resolved by lowering the dose, but this will invariably lead to a corresponding decrease in the control of motor symptoms. In some cases the dosage of levodopa can be maintained, but the postural hypotension prevented by administration of fludrocortisone. The patient's sodium intake has to be sufficient for fludrocortisone to be effective. Doses higher than 0.2 mg have been used, but this increases the risk of heart failure especially in the elderly. Hypokalaemia may occur, necessitating the use of potassium supplements.

Midodrine produces peripheral vasoconstriction and consequently helps maintain blood pressure. It is a sympathomimetic with selective alpha-agonist activity. Dosage is usually commenced at 2.5 mg two or three times daily and gradually increased until effective up to a maximum of 10 mg three times daily. Midodrine is not marketed in the UK, but is obtained by some hospitals from sources abroad. It is important to ensure that the drug therapy for postural hypotension does not result in supine hypertension.

Problems with sleeping

Abnormal movements and sometimes tremor can clearly lead to disturbed sleep, not only for the patient but also a bed partner. Although in the majority of patients it is these symptoms which are responsible for poor sleep, other conditions such as restless leg syndrome (RLS) may prevent good sleep. Symptoms of RLS may be reduced with levodopa, and the directly acting dopamine agonists may also decrease the severity of symptoms.

In a small number of patients with Parkinson's disease, a condition known as rapid eye movement (REM) sleep behaviour disorder (RBD) can occur. In these cases, the patient makes movements in line with a dream they are having.

It is important to correctly identify with the patient the true cause of insomnia. When it is due to physical symptoms such as abnormal movement, tremor, muscle cramp, RLS or nightmares, it is usually quite obvious and the patient can describe the key issue preventing sleep. However, underlying anxiety or depression (see previous) may be less obvious and may not be readily apparent as the cause. Both anxiety and depression can be effectively treated with appropriate therapy, not only making the patient happier in themselves but also improving quality of sleep, which in turn results in the patient feeling less tired during the daytime and more inclined to exercise. Carrying out more activities during the day is of great benefit to the patient, both physically and mentally. It is therefore very important that sleep problems are identified and treated in the most effective way to improve overall patient wellbeing. The management of sleep disturbance rightly receives thorough coverage in the guideline published in 2006,[13] the key recommendations of which are outlined in Chapter 8 (page 156). Daytime hypersomnolence has become increasingly recognised as a significant problem for patients with Parkinson's disease, sometimes leading to sudden onset of sleep. Clinical trials with modafinil have generally produced disappointing results, though one study showed a useful effect as assessed using the Epworth Sleepiness Scale (ESS).[14] Nocturnal akinesia, where the patient finds they are unable to turn over in bed, can substantially reduce sleep, in turn increasing the likelihood of daytime hypersomnolence. Modified-release levodopa products may be helpful; the long-acting dopamine agonist cabergoline has also been used for this problem.

Sexual problems

Sexual problems may occur due to difficulties arising from the physical symptoms of Parkinson's disease or other symptoms such as depression. Movement disorders can clearly affect sexual activity, especially where mobility is compromised. Optimising treatment of these symptoms with anti-Parkinson's drugs may be all that is necessary to improve the situation. If depression and/or anxiety are a feature of a patient's condition, these should be addressed in any case, and this in itself may solve or at least reduce sexual problems. However, it should be remembered that some antidepressant drugs and anxiolytics can themselves cause adverse effects on sexual function. In cases of impotence or where bladder symptoms may be contributing to the problem, referral to a urologist or gynaecologist should be considered as appropriate. It should be noted that levodopa and dopamine agonists can markedly increase sexual drive, an effect not due solely to an improvement in mobility.

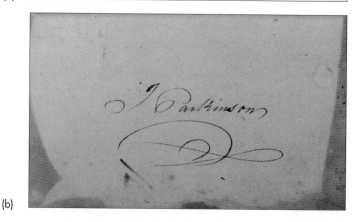

Plate 1 **(a)** Title page of James Parkinson's *An Essay on the Shaking Palsy;* **(b)** no pictures of James Parkinson have been located, however his signature is on documentation held in The Royal London Hospital's Museum. Pictures courtesy of Jonathan Evans, Royal London Hospital Archives.

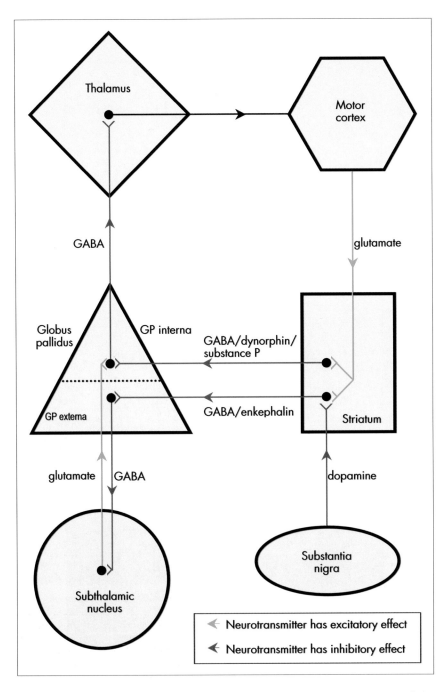

Plate 2 Diagrammatic representation showing key neuronal pathways of the basal ganglia potentially involved in Parkinson's disease.

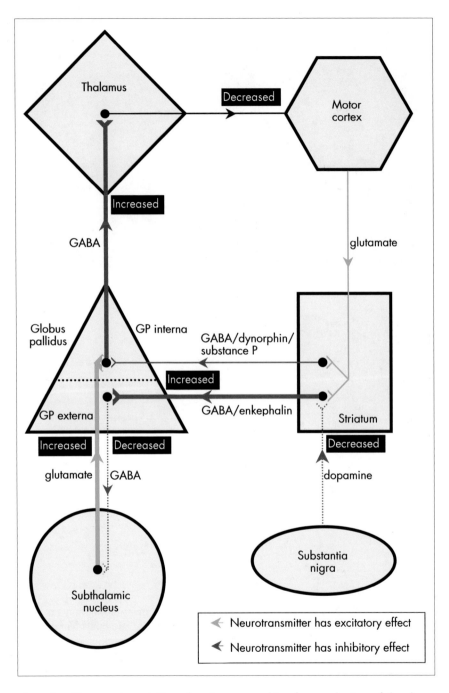

Plate 3 Changes in activities of pathways resulting from reduction of the dopaminergic input from the substantia nigra caused by Parkinson's disease.

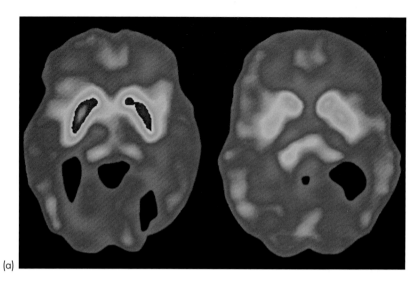

(a)

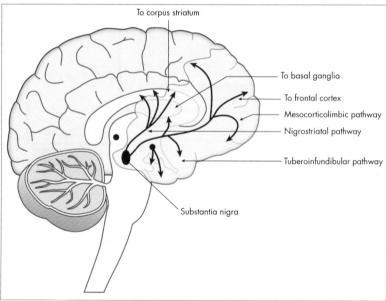

To corpus striatum

To basal ganglia

To frontal cortex

Mesocorticolimbic pathway

Nigrostriatal pathway

Tuberoinfundibular pathway

Substantia nigra

(b)

Plate 4 **(a)** Positron emission tomography (PET) can give information on brain function, compared to CT and MRI scans which provide anatomical images. A positron-emitting radioactive isotope is tagged to the molecule of interest, which is then administered to the patient. ^{18}F-6-fluorodopa (^{18}F-dopa) is used to show dopa uptake and conversion to dopamine in the nigrostriatal dopaminergic neurons. The image on the right shows the loss of dopamine neurons in the brain of a person with Parkinson's disease. **(b)** Dopamine pathways in the human brain. Pictures courtesy of Schwarz Pharma Ltd.

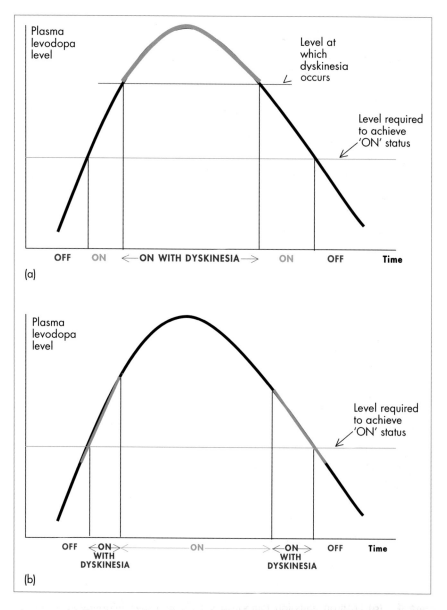

Plate 5 **(a)** Illustration of peak-dose dyskinesia and **(b)** biphasic dyskinesia.

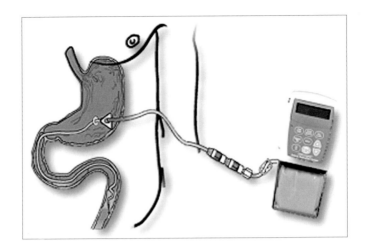

Plate 6 Diagram showing the system for the administration of duodopa.

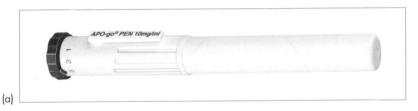

(a)

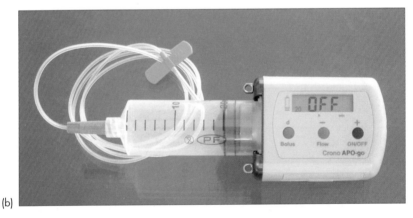

(b)

Plate 7 **(a)** Apomorphine injections can be given with a pen device (APO-go Pen). These are suitable when the number of injections needed each day does not exceed ten. **(b)** The apomorphine infusion pump (Crono APO-go Pump). This is used when patients have a large number of 'off' periods each day making repeated injections impractical. The pump is programmed to deliver the dosage best suited for the patient. Pictures courtesy of Britannia Pharmaceuticals Ltd.

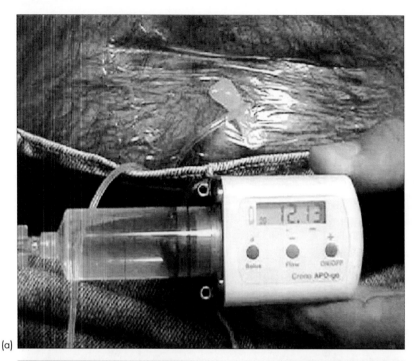

(a)

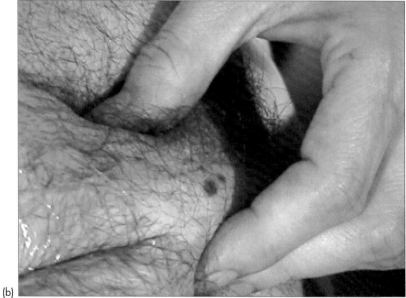

(b)

Plate 8 **(a)** The apomorphine pump is connected to a butterfly cannula which is sited each day in the abdomen (as shown) or the subcutaneous tissue of the thigh. **(b)** Apomorphine can cause injection-site reactions including nodule formation. Pictures courtesy of Britannia Pharmaceuticals Ltd.

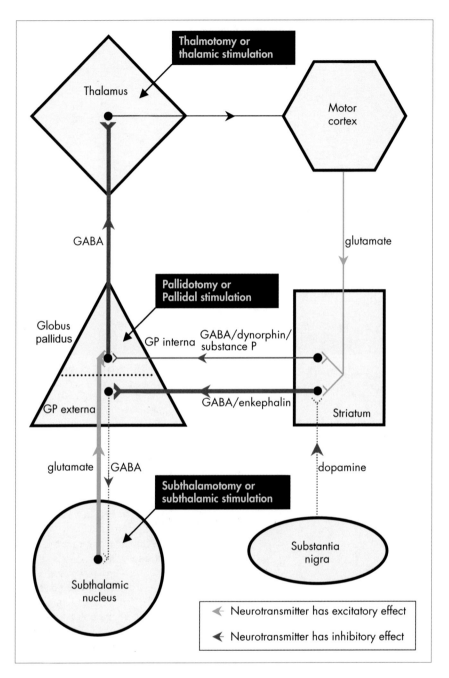

Plate 9 Sites for lesioning or deep brain stimulation in patients with Parkinson's disease.

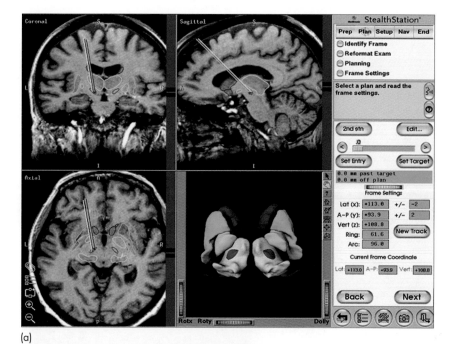

(a)

(b)

Plate 10 **(a)** A computer-generated image which assists in planning the implantation trajectory of the lead for deep brain stimulation (DBS). The computer software (FrameLink from Medtronic) facilitates stereotactic surgical planning and intra-operative control. The images allow accurate determination of the burr hole entry point in relation to the target, and help ensure the ventricles and blood vessels are missed. **(b)** The stimulator device and leads which pass the electrical current to the electrode(s) implanted into the appropriate area of the brain. The device itself is implanted under the skin normally below the collar bone (see Plate 11). The picture also shows the unit. Both pictures reproduced with permission from Medtronic®.

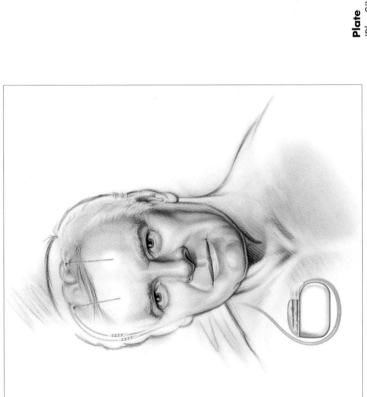

Plate 11 Position of bilateral electrodes and the stimulator device for deep brain stimulation. Reproduced with permission from Medtronic®.

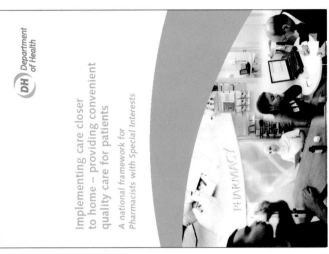

Plate 12 Establishing pharmacists with special interests (PhwSI) in primary care provides an opportunity for pharmacists to specialise in conditions such as Parkinson's disease and increase patient access to support with their drug therapy. The Department of Health published details in September 2006.

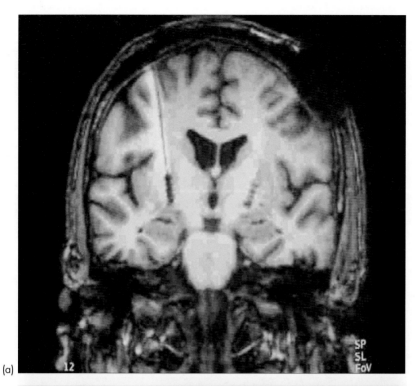

(a)

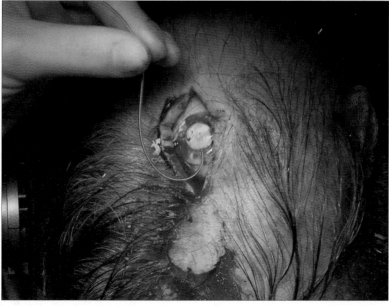

(b)

Plate 13 **(a)** Implanted electrodes for deep brain stimulation. **(b)** Lead fixation prior to closing the surgical incision. Both pictures reproduced with permission from Medtronic®.

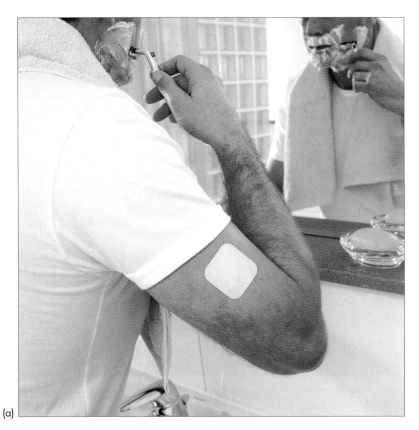

(a)

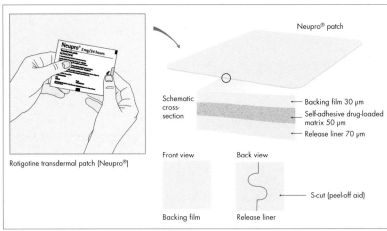

(b)

Plate 14 New routes for administering drugs used to treat Parkinson's disease are continually being explored. A transdermal patch delivering the dopamine agonist rotigotine (Neupro) was launched in the UK by Schwarz in 2006. Pictures courtesy of Schwarz Pharma Ltd.

For men with sexual problems such as erectile dysfunction, a number of drugs are now available which can prove very effective. Sildenafil, tadalafil and vardenafil are drugs which have become available in recent years and have revolutionised the management of erectile dysfunction. They inhibit the enzyme phosphodiesterase type-5 resulting in improved blood flow in the penis and hence a sustained erection. Side-effects such as headache, flushing, dizziness and dyspepsia can occur, and there have been cases of priapism and hypersensitivity reactions. Back pain and myalgia have been reported with tadalafil and vardenafil. Phosphodiesterase type-5 inhibitors should not be taken by patients with unstable angina, or a history of recent stroke or myocardial infarction. Further details of these three drugs are given in Focus on treatments for erectile dysfunction (6.1). In the UK, prescribing these drugs on the NHS is only allowed for certain groups of patients. Fortunately, patients suffering with Parkinson's disease are specifically included on the list.

FOCUS ON TREATMENTS FOR ERECTILE DYSFUNCTION 6.1

Phosphodiesterase type-5 inhibitors used to treat erectile dysfunction

NB: Parkinson's disease is specifically listed as a condition for which these drugs may be prescribed in the UK on the NHS.

Sildenafil

Dosage

- Initially 50 mg approximately 1 h before sexual activity
- Subsequent doses should be adjusted according to response – between 25 mg and 100 mg
- No more than one dose should be taken in 24 h
- A single dose of 100 mg should not be exceeded

Notes

- *Food*: if taken with food, the onset of action may be delayed.

Preparations

- Tablets of 25 mg sildenafil (as citrate) (Viagra)
- Tablets of 50 mg sildenafil (as citrate) (Viagra)
- Tablets of 100 mg sildenafil (as citrate) (Viagra)

continued overleaf

Focus on treatments for erectile dysfunction 6.1 (continued)

Tadalafil

Dosage

- Initially 10 mg approximately half an hour before sexual activity
- Subsequent doses should be adjusted if necessary according to response – either 10 mg or 20 mg
- No more than one dose should be taken in 24 h
- A single dose of 20 mg should not be exceeded

Notes

- *Duration of action*: in some patients the effect can persist for 24 h or more.

Preparations

- Tablets of 10 mg tadalafil (Cialis)
- Tablets of 20 mg tadalafil (Cialis)

Vardenafil

Dosage

- Initially 10 mg approximately half an hour to an hour before sexual activity
- Subsequent doses should be adjusted if necessary according to response – between 5 mg and 20 mg
- No more than one dose should be taken in 24 h
- A single dose of 20 mg should not be exceeded

Notes

- *Elderly patients*: the initial dosage should be reduced to 5 mg in elderly patients.
- *Food*: if taken with high-fat food, the onset of action may be delayed.

Preparations

- Tablets of 5 mg vardenafil (as hydrochloride trihydrate) (Levitra)
- Tablets of 10 mg vardenafil (as hydrochloride trihydrate) (Levitra)
- Tablets of 20 mg vardenafil (as hydrochloride trihydrate) (Levitra)

The phosphodiesterase type-5 inhibitors potentially interact with a number of other drugs. The hypotensive effects of nitrates, alpha-blockers, calcium channel blockers such as nifedipine, and the potassium channel activator nicorandil can be increased by phosphodiesterase type-5 inhibitors. Certain antibacterials (e.g. erythromycin), antifungal agents (e.g. ketoconazole, itraconazole) and antivirals (e.g. ritonavir, saquinavir) may increase the levels of phosphodiesterase type-5 inhibitors, increasing the risk of adverse effects. Interactions with a number of other drugs and with grapefruit juice are possible.

References

1. Chaudhuri KR, Healy DG, Schapira AH. Non-motor symptoms of Parkinson's disease: diagnosis and management. *Lancet Neurol* 2006; 5: 235–245.
2. Lauterbach EC. The neuropsychiatry of Parkinson's disease and related disorders. *Psychiatr Clin North Am* 2004; 27: 801–825.
3. Miyasaki JM, Shannon K, Voon V, *et al.* Practice parameter: evaluation and treatment of depression, psychosis, and dementia in Parkinson disease (an evidence-based review): report of the Quality Standards Subcommittee of the American Academy of Neurology. *Neurology* 2006; 66: 996–1002.
4. Hyson HC, Johnson AM, Jog MS. Sublingual atropine for sialorrhea secondary to parkinsonism: a pilot study. *Mov Disord* 2002; 17: 1318.
5. Goetz CG, Koller WC, Poewe W, *et al.* Treatment of depression in idiopathic Parkinson's disease. *Mov Disord* 2002; 17 (Suppl 4): S112–S119.
6. Jiménez-Jiménez FJ, Tejeiro J, Martinez-Junquera G, *et al.* Parkinsonism exacerbated by paroxetine. *Neurology* 1994; 44: 2406.
7. Weintraub D, Morales KH, Moberg PJ, *et al.* Antidepressant studies in Parkinson's disease: a review and meta-analysis. *Mov Disord* 2005; 20: 1161–1169.
8. Wint DP, Okun MS, Fernandez HH. Psychosis in Parkinson's disease. *J Geriatr Psychiatry Neurol* 2004; 17: 127–136.
9. Maidment I, Fox C, Boustani M. Cholinesterase inhibitors for Parkinson's disease dementia (Cochrane Review). *Cochrane Database Syst Rev* 2006 Jan 25; (1): CD004747.
10. Emre M, Aarsland D, Albanese A, *et al.* Rivastigmine for dementia associated with Parkinson's disease. *N Engl J Med* 2004; 351: 2509–2518.
11. Ravina B, Putt M, Siderowf A, *et al.* Donepezil for dementia in Parkinson's disease: a randomised, double blind, placebo controlled, crossover study. *J Neurol Neurosurg Psychiatry* 2005; 76: 934–939.
12. Aarsland D, Hutchinson M, Larsen JP. Cognitive, psychiatric and motor response to galantamine in Parkinson's disease with dementia. *Int J Geriatr Psychiatry* 2003; 18: 937–941.
13. National Collaborating Centre for Chronic Conditions. *Parkinson's Disease: diagnosis and management in primary and secondary care* [full guideline]. London: National Collaborating Centre for Chronic Conditions, 2006, 124–128.
14. Adler CH, Caviness JN, Hentz JG, *et al.* Randomized trial of modafinil for treating subjective daytime sleepiness in patients with Parkinson's disease. *Mov Disord* 2003; 18: 287–293.

Further reading

Aarsland D, Andersen K, Larsen JP, *et al.* Prevalence and characteristics of dementia in Parkinson's disease: an 8 year prospective study. *Arch Neurol* 2003; 60: 387–392.

Allcock LM, Ullyart K, Kenny R, *et al.* Frequency of orthostatic hypotension in a community acquired cohort of patients with Parkinson's disease. *J Neurol Neurosurg Psychiatry* 2003; 75: 1470–1471.

Giladi N, Shabtai H, Gurevich T, *et al.* Rivastigmine (Exelon) for dementia in patients with Parkinson's disease. *Acta Neurol Scand* 2003; 108: 368–373.

Leentjens AFG. Depression in Parkinson's disease: conceptual issues and clinical challenges. *J Geriatr Psychiatry Neurol* 2004; 17:120–126.

Leroi I, Brandt J, Reich S, *et al.* Randomized placebo-controlled trial of donepezil in cognitive impairment in Parkinson's disease. *Int J Geriatr Psychiatry* 2004; 19: 1–8.

McKeith IG, Mosimann UP. Dementia with Lewy bodies and Parkinson's disease. *Parkinsonism Relat Disord* 2004; 10 (Suppl): 15–18.

Montgomery EB. Rehabilitative approaches to Parkinson's disease. *Parkinsonism Relat Disord* 2004; 10 (Suppl 1): S43–47.

7

Developments and future treatments

There has been a massive search over many years to find new agents to improve upon the drugs available for treating Parkinson's disease. Often research efforts have focused on drugs within the same pharmacological class as existing treatments in an attempt to improve on efficacy or reduce side-effects (e.g. the dopamine agonists). In some cases, different ways of formulating or administering drugs already widely used have been examined (e.g. the intra-duodenal administration of co-careldopa gel). In recent years, a number of new drugs have become available; the two non-ergolinic dopamine agonists, pramipexole and ropinirole in the second half of the 1990s and rasagiline in 2005, a monoamine oxidase-B inhibitor which joins selegiline, which until then was the only drug in this class used in Parkinson's disease. More recently in 2006 rotigotine was launched, another non-ergolinic dopamine agonist, but this time administered via a transdermal delivery system in the form of a patch which the patient applies each day (see Plate 14).

Many researchers have moved away from the existing pharmacological approaches and have sought therapies that work through different mechanisms. Often this has been driven by the increased understanding we have of the pathophysiology of Parkinson's disease. Alternative receptor sites and neurotransmitters have been the focus of intense research in the quest for better therapies (e.g. adenosine A_2A receptor antagonists). There is growing evidence that the non-physiological stimulation of dopamine receptors with the drugs currently available is actually responsible for some of the complications that occur with levodopa therapy and disease progression. The pulsatile stimulation of dopamine receptors does not closely mimic the normal state of physiological stimulation and is thought to adversely affect glutamate and other receptors. The firing pattern of neurons is regulated at both pre- and postsynaptic levels, and ways of influencing these mechanisms are being studied. Attention is being focused on synaptic vesicle proteins and non-synaptic gap junction communication systems. Drugs which can influence the phosphorylation state of N-methyl-D-aspartate

(NMDA) receptors by affecting signal transduction systems may also be developed. Not only are these efforts addressing the need for improvements in the management of the symptoms of Parkinson's disease, which is all that existing drugs are able to do, but ways of delaying the progression of the disease, or even reversing the disease process, or preventing it in the first place, have been subjected to extensive research.

Other areas of research have centred on 'repairing' the damage occurring in the brain. One example is the use of glial cell line-derived neurotrophic factor (GDNF) to hopefully restore neural function and induce 'neural sprouting' to replace degenerated cells. Gene therapy is also receiving much attention. Clearly the problem is being approached from many different angles in the desire to make a major breakthrough and offer more effective treatments to patients. In many cases, research into possible treatments for other neurodegenerative diseases such as motor neuron disease, multiple sclerosis, and Alzheimer's disease has provided new ideas for the treatment of Parkinson's disease, and vice versa.

Enormous efforts are being made in the quest to find better treatments for neurological conditions, and rightly so. However, in parallel with this it is also right that we fully optimise the benefits that can be derived from those drugs we already have, by assessing new regimens, combinations and the ways in which they are used. This chapter gives an overview of the main approaches being explored and cites examples of new agents that are being assessed for their clinical value.

Drugs affecting dopaminergic function

Natural sources of levodopa

The list of complementary therapies on page 87 (Box 4.1) includes Ayurveda, the ancient Indian healing system which combines changes in lifestyle, diet, exercise, meditation and the use of herbal remedies such as extracts prepared from the seeds of the mucuna plant. A double-blind clinical trial has been carried out at The National Hospital for Neurology and Neurosurgery (London) comparing the effects of co-careldopa (levodopa plus carbidopa) with those of a preparation made from the plant *Mucuna pruriens*.[1] The mucuna preparation produced an onset of effect twice as fast as the co-careldopa treatment (34.6 min compared to 68.5 min respectively). The mean 'on' time was more than half an hour longer (37 min) following administration of the mucuna preparation. Tolerability and the occurrence of dyskinesia were similar for both treatments. The authors concluded that the natural source of levodopa may have clinical advantages over the form currently used in medical practice, and believe further randomised studies should be carried out to see if the initial findings in this rather small study are confirmed.

Esters of levodopa

The methyl ester form of levodopa, known as melevodopa is highly water soluble. After oral administration it can decrease the time to achieve the 'on' phase and may produce a more stable clinical effect. Further work is needed to confirm any benefits over existing levodopa preparations. An ethyl ester of levodopa, known as etilevodopa has also been produced. This has greater gastric solubility and recent trial results in patients with Parkinson's disease showed theoretical advantages in terms of the pharmacokinetics of etilevodopa. Unfortunately, no meaningful differences were shown in time to achieve the 'on' phase or other clinical measures.[2]

Dopamine agonists

In 2006, the first skin patch was launched for treating Parkinson's disease. This delivers the dopamine agonist rotigotine via the trans-dermal route. Studies are also under way with the dopamine agonist lysuride to see whether this can be administered in a similar way. The intranasal route is also being assessed for administering some dopamine agonists including apomorphine (page 55) and rotigotine.

The search for new dopamine agonists offering advantages over those currently available has been in progress for many years. The relevance of the selectivity for specific dopamine receptors is still unclear. Sumanirole is a novel dopamine agonist since it is highly selective for the dopamine D_2 subtype of receptors. It has reached Phase III clinical trials in patients with Parkinson's disease, but early results suggest it has no advantages over established drugs in this class. SLV-308 is being assessed and is not only a partial D_2 agonist, but also possesses 5-hydroxytryptamine $(5\text{-HT})_{1A}$ agonist properties. ACP-103 has partial agonist actions on both dopamine D_2 and D_3 receptors; it also has effects on 5-HT_{2A} receptors and is an acetylcholine M_1 receptor agonist. Studies are proceeding to assess the effect of ACP-103 in Parkinson's patients suffering with treatment-induced psychosis. The drug is also being tested as adjunctive therapy in schizophrenia. BP-897 is a partial agonist of dopamine D_3 receptors, and in laboratory animals has been found to substantially reduce the severity of dyskinesia resulting from levodopa treatment, without affecting motor improvement. Piribedil is a D_2/D_3 dopamine agonist with additional α_2-noradrenergic properties. It has been licensed for use in some countries (not the UK) for the treatment of Parkinson's disease, both as monotherapy and in combination with levodopa. Research into other dopamine agonists continues, but it is unlikely they will offer substantial advantages over those already in use.

A considerable amount of work has taken place to determine whether dopamine agonists have neuroprotective effects. Although *in vitro* and animal studies suggest such an effect, there is little evidence so far that neuroprotection occurs in Parkinson's disease. Several methodological problems have been identified with the clinical studies that have looked at any potential neuroprotective effects that ropinirole and pramipexole may have.[3]

Monoamine oxidase type-B inhibitors

A number of agents have been developed that inhibit monoamine oxidase (MAO)-B, but apart from rasagiline, there have not been any new ones brought into clinical use since selegiline. Safinamide inhibits MAO-B and additionally antagonises calcium and sodium channels. It has been studied for its effects on Parkinson's disease and it appears to produce a small improvement in symptoms. Work is proceeding to see whether it has a neuroprotective effect as has been claimed by some people for the current drugs in this class. So far, studies that are of long enough duration, and that contain sufficient numbers of patients to scientifically show any neuroprotective value in Parkinson's disease, have not been forthcoming.

Catechol-O-methyltransferase inhibitors

At present, the only catechol-O-methyltransferase (COMT) inhibitor in routine use for treating Parkinson's disease is entacapone, though tolcapone is available for use in certain circumstances. A new compound known as BIA-3202 has been tested in humans and shown to reduce COMT activity in erythrocytes. Whether further work will produce encouraging results in clinical terms remains to be seen.

Monoamine reuptake inhibitors

Much research has taken place assessing the potential of agents which block the reuptake of monoamines. Brasofensine (BMS-204756) is described as a dopamine transporter antagonist and has been assessed in patients with Parkinson's disease who are receiving co-careldopa.[4] Unfortunately results were disappointing and motor function was not significantly improved.

Enhanced dopamine synthesis

Although only recently licensed in the UK, the anti-epileptic drug zonisamide has been available for a number of years in other countries. The suggestion that it may have beneficial effects in Parkinson's disease was made in 2001 by researchers in Japan when a 300 mg dose was given to a patient who had both Parkinson's disease and convulsions.[5] Not only did the frequency of convulsions reduce, but the patient experienced a dramatic improvement in their symptoms of Parkinson's disease. Further work assessing the value of zonisamide in Parkinson's disease was subsequently carried out and a multicentre, randomised, double-blind trial published in 2007.[6] The results of this showed that when used as adjunctive therapy in patients showing insufficient response to levodopa (plus peripheral dopa decarboxylase inhibitor), significant improvements occurred in motor fluctuations, dyskinesias and tremor. Patients given zonisamide 25 mg or 50 mg had significant benefit as measured using the Unified Parkinson's Disease Rating Scale (UPDRS) – Part III (motor examination). It was also found that the frequency of dyskinesia decreased in the group of patients taking zonisamide 50 mg. Zonisamide produced no significant changes in parts I, II and IV of the UPDRS. The doses used in this study were much lower than those typically used to treat epilepsy, suggesting that the mechanism of action in Parkinson's disease is different from that for epilepsy. Zonisamide has many pharmacological effects including inhibition of MAO-B, and for some time it was this property which was considered to be responsible, at least in part, for its beneficial effects in Parkinson's disease. However it is now felt that the main mechanism of action of zonisamide in Parkinson's disease is an increase in dopamine synthesis. It has been proposed that this results from the drug increasing tyrosine hydroxylase activity and tyrosine hydroxylase messenger RNA.

Drugs affecting non-dopaminergic pathways

Alpha$_2$-adrenergic receptor antagonists

Fipamezole (JP-1730)

Fipamezole belongs to a new class of drugs being investigated for their effectiveness in Parkinson's disease. It acts on α_2-adrenergic receptors and is found in animal models of Parkinson's disease to prolong the duration of action of levodopa and reduce the severity of dyskinesia.[7] These benefits have been replicated in a study carried out in patients with advanced Parkinson's disease.[8] Although adverse effects included pallor, nausea, sweating and dizziness, fipamezole did not produce significant effects on the cardiovascular system. Further studies are needed to confirm these preliminary results and ascertain the value of fipamezole in clinical practice.

Adenosine A$_2$A receptor antagonists

Several different adenosine receptors have been identified in the brain and it is thought that adenosine affects the activity of certain nerve cells. Neurobiological studies have shown that a subset of adenosine receptors known as adenosine A_2A is present in the striatum, and it has been suggested that these modulate the effect of dopamine as well as interacting with other receptors such as those for glutamate and GABA. The pharmacological approach of blocking A_2A receptors has been the subject of much enthusiastic research in recent years. Agents that block these receptors may reduce some of the adverse effects that occur with levodopa therapy, such as dyskinesia. It has also been hypothesised that blocking adenosine A_2A receptors can have a neuroprotective effect on dopaminergic pathways. More than 2000 chemicals have been synthesised and screened for adenosine A_2A antagonist properties, and there is cautious anticipation that this will be a successful new pharmacological approach to the treatment of Parkinson's disease. Studies are also under way to see whether adenosine A_2A antagonists have useful therapeutic effects in other neurodegenerative disorders.

Istradefylline (KW-6002)

Istradefylline is probably the adenosine A_2A receptor antagonist which has generated most enthusiasm from researchers. Animal studies suggest that this agent can improve motor function without causing dyskinesia.[9]

Tremor is also improved. The limited experience gained from human studies supports these findings. Patients receiving low-dose levodopa together with the adenosine A_2A antagonist istradefylline, seem to achieve the same degree of clinical improvement in their symptoms as taking levodopa alone at optimised dosage, but without the same extent of dyskinesia.[10] Other studies have produced variable results when looking at the time patients spend in the 'off' state, some showing a significant reduction in this, others failing to do so. A clinical trial using istradefylline in advanced Parkinson's disease failed to show improvement of dyskinesia when used in levodopa-treated patients, but 'on' time was significantly increased as reflected in the patients' home diaries, though no difference was found between the drug and placebo using the UPDRS or Clinical Global Impression of Change.[11] The drug was well tolerated, nausea being the most commonly reported problem. A Japanese company submitted a new drug application for istradefylline to the US Food and Drug Administration (FDA) during 2007; this is still awaiting approval.

Other A_2A receptor antagonists

Theophylline also blocks adenosine A_2A receptors and is being studied to determine whether it may produce useful effects in Parkinson's disease.

Caffeine blocks adenosine A_2A receptors, but not so actively as the drugs above. However, this provides a degree of rationale to the belief by some that tea and coffee can be helpful in controlling the symptoms of Parkinson's disease.

AMPA receptor antagonists

AMPA (alpha-amino-3-hydroxy-5-methyl-4-isoxazole-propionic acid) antagonists represent a new approach to the management of Parkinson's disease. Talampanel is the first drug in the class to be studied in humans and it is considered it might be useful in decreasing the problems of dyskinesia.

Neuronal synchronisation modulators

Many anti-epileptic agents work by changing the ability of cells to discharge rapidly, repetitively or synchronously. At a molecular level, it is believed these effects can influence mood, pain and movement disorders such as dyskinesia and tremor. This in part explains the therapeutic value of the anti-epileptic drugs such as carbamazepine and sodium valproate in the management of bipolar disorder. Research into the potentially useful effects of anti-epileptic drugs in controlling the symptoms of Parkinson's disease has so far focused on levetiracetam which has an action described as a neuronal synchronisation modulator. The mechanism by which this effect is produced is unknown, though it has been shown that agents such as levetiracetam bind to the synaptic vesicle protein SV2A,[12] and this possibly affects the transmission of impulses in pathways affected by Parkinson's disease. Some animal studies have also shown an effect on striatal GABAergic transmission.[13]

Levetiracetam

The relatively new anti-epileptic drug levetiracetam has been assessed in Parkinson's disease following initial encouraging results from animal studies. The results of studies in patients suffering with essential tremor have been disappointing, as have the results in Parkinson's disease when looking at the onset of dyskinesia following *do novo* treatment with levodopa. However the results in patients receiving a combination of levodopa plus levetiracetam following a 'drug holiday' are more encouraging. In these cases levetiracetam appeared to reduce the problem of levodopa-induced dyskinesia. It has been postulated that previous treatment with levetiracetam can modify the mechanisms involved in the development of dyskinesia. This may result from altering the 'priming phenomenon', which is thought to be allied to long-term changes occurring in synaptic function that are responsible for the dyskinesia seen in Parkinson's disease.

In a small pilot study of nine patients suffering with substantial levodopa-induced dyskinesia, levetiracetam increased the proportion of time that patients spent in the 'on' phase without troublesome dyskinesia.[14] The efficacy of levodopa in treating the symptoms of Parkinson's disease was not compromised by the levetiracetam. The dosage used was increased from 250 mg per day up to 3 g per day, and unfortunately somnolence was a common side-effect. Five of the nine patients dropped out of the study because of either this adverse effect, reduced alertness, or dizziness and confusion.

Other drugs that bind to synaptic vesicle protein 2A ligand include brivaracetam and seletracetam. These are potential treatments for neurological conditions such as epilepsy and neuropathic pain, and possibly Parkinson's disease.

5-hydroxytryptamine (5-HT)$_{1A}$ agonists

Motor dysfunction seen in advanced Parkinson's disease may in part be due to intermittent stimulation of dopamine receptors in the striatum. When severe denervation of the dopaminergic pathway has occurred, exogenous levodopa is mainly converted to dopamine in serotonergic nerve terminals. It has been suggested that 5-HT$_{1A}$ autoreceptors control both serotonin and dopamine release. Inhibiting serotonergic neuron firing in the striatum of patients with Parkinson's disease may preserve physiological intrasynaptic dopamine levels, which in turn may reduce fluctuations in motor function and dyskinesias.

Sarizotan

Sarizotan is a selective 5-HT$_{1A}$ agonist which has been assessed in patients with advanced Parkinson's disease.[15] Sarizotan had little effect on the severity of symptoms in Parkinson's disease, but was found to decrease levodopa-induced dyskinesia and prolong the duration of action of levodopa. Further studies will show whether sarizotan is likely to be of clinical value as adjunctive therapy with levodopa.

Cannabinoids

The effectiveness of cannabinoids in treating various neurological conditions including multiple sclerosis, neuropathic pain and spasticity, has been the subject of much research for many years. A number of these patients resort to marijuana and are likely to continue to do so until medicinal cannabinoids are more readily available for therapeutic use. One study carried out by an academic pharmacy department of a university in Czech republic, showed that one-quarter of patients with Parkinson's disease attending a movement disorder clinic had taken cannabis. Of these, nearly one-half claimed to have derived benefit in their motor symptoms from doing so.[16] Sativex (delta-9-tetrahydro-cannabiol 2.92 mg/actuation + cannabidiol 2.7 mg/actuation oro-mucosal spray) is now available in some countries including the UK, but not specifically licensed for use in Parkinson's disease. One of the most studied cannabinoids is delta-9-tetrahydrocannabinol (THC); this is also the most active compound of the several hundred constituents present in marijuana.

The globus pallidus and the substantia nigra are known to have a high presence of cannabinoid receptors. Since these areas of the brain are involved in the control of movement, it is feasible that cannabinoids could produce a useful effect by relieving some of the symptoms of Parkinson's disease. There is some evidence that these receptors influence the activity of certain neuronal pathways, including increasing GABAergic transmission, decreasing glutamate release and modifying dopaminergic uptake.[17] It has even been suggested that changes in endogenous cannabinoid activity may play a part in the pathophysiology of neurological conditions such as Parkinson's disease.

Unfortunately, as is the case for a number of studies of cannabinoids in neurological conditions, the scientific evidence supporting the use of cannabinoids in Parkinson's disease is lacking. A randomised, double-blind, placebo-controlled study examining the value of cannabis in patients with Parkinson's disease produced disappointing results.[18] Although cannabis was well tolerated, no useful effect was obtained in any of the outcome measures including dyskinesia scores, and patient assessments of activities of daily living and quality-of-life scales. The authors concluded that cannabis failed to show any benefit in either objective or subjective measures of dyskinesias or symptoms of Parkinson's disease.

Glutamate antagonists

Amantadine, a drug which has been in use for many years for treating Parkinson's disease, is known to reduce the effects of glutamate by blocking NMDA receptors. Claims have been made that the drug can slow progression of the disease by reducing the extent of cell death caused by excess glutamate activity. Although there is no good evidence for this, research into new agents that block NMDA receptors continues. Riluzole, a drug used to treat amyotrophic lateral sclerosis (a form of motor neuron disease), is thought to block presynaptic release of glutamate and influence the postsynaptic effects of the transmitter. However, the results of a trial with riluzole in early Parkinson's disease were disappointing.[19] Other agents which are being assessed include remacemide, bupidine and rimantadine, which is a derivative of amantadine possessing a longer duration of action.

Nicotine receptor agonists

It has been known for a long time that the risk of developing Parkinson's disease in people who smoke seems to be lower than in those that do not. Although it is an assumption, the conclusion has been made that stimulation of nicotine receptors somehow conveys a degree of protection, although the use of nicotine patches does not appear to be effective. Stimulation of certain types of nicotine receptors in the brain is thought to influence the release of neurotransmitters including dopamine and acetylcholine. Work is still at an early stage, but a number of compounds have been tested including SIB-1508Y and ABT-418. The possibility that agents such as these may improve memory is also being explored.

Neuroprotective/neurorestorative agents

Antioxidants

A number of terms are used to describe various forms of neuroprotection. 'Neuroprotection' itself signifies a reduction in the rate of deterioration due to interventions that modify the pathophysiology of Parkinson's disease. 'Neurorescue' is a term used to describe the salvage of dying neurons, thus maintaining the level of functioning cells. 'Neurorestoration', as the term implies, results in an increase in neurons. At present, the main avenues for this development are the use of nerve growth factor or cell implantation.

The products resulting from the oxidation of dopamine are thought to be toxic to dopaminergic neurons. Many people have claimed that inhibitors of MAO such as selegiline not only helped maintain the levels of dopamine, but also had neuroprotective properties by blocking the oxidation of dopamine. Any evidence that this happens in practice is very weak. Whether evidence will be forthcoming showing neuroprotective effects of other MAO inhibitors such as rasagiline is uncertain; many people think it is unlikely. Antioxidants have received much attention for their possible effects on the progression of Parkinson's disease, but most studies with compounds such as vitamin E and vitamin C have been disappointing. One study looking at 2-year follow-up data failed to demonstrate that vitamin E reduced the need to commence treatment with levodopa or had useful effects as measured with a number of rating scales (see also page 89).[20] Neuroprotection and neurorestoration therapies, which slow or stop, or even reverse disease progression, are the subject of much ongoing research. Many agents have shown promise in the laboratory setting, but establishing clear clinical endpoints that can be used in clinical trials is very difficult.[21] Differentiating between symptomatic effects and any contribution due to neuroprotection remains a challenge.

Anti-apoptotic kinase inhibitors

The process of apoptosis has been described as cell suicide. If the genes that trigger this process can be blocked, the apoptosis of dopamine cells may be inhibited. CEP-1347, described as a mixed lineage kinase inhibitor, has this effect. In an animal model of Parkinson's disease it seems to improve dopaminergic neuron survival;[22] however, hopes that these results can be replicated in humans are fading.

Glial cell line-derived neurotrophic factor (GDNF)

There is good evidence that laboratory animals with an induced form of Parkinson's disease recover from damage to the dopamine neurons when treated with GDNF. This protein is thought to protect and restore neuronal pathways and increase the production of dopamine. Several studies have been carried out where GDNF has been administered to patients with Parkinson's disease through a small catheter implanted into the posterior putamen. A paper published by researchers in Bristol claims that substantial improvement in motor function and activities of daily living is achieved with no serious side-effects and no impairment of cognition.[23] Similar results were reported in a study from the US, following the intra-putaminal infusion of GDNF.[24] The intra-putaminal catheter was implanted on the opposite side to that most affected by Parkinson's disease. GDNF was infused at 2-month intervals. Significant improvement in symptoms such as balance, gait and speed of hand movements occurred bilaterally. Scores on the UPDRS were significantly improved. The authors concluded that the unilateral administration of GDNF produced significant, sustained bilateral effects. However, work carried out in Canada appears to contradict these positive results.[25] This randomised controlled trial was carried out in 34 patients (a larger number than in the two studies above). No significant difference was found in any of the UPDRS scores between patients who received doses of GDNF and those who received placebo. This negative clinical outcome resulted, despite ^{18}F-dopa influx. The disappointing results from the Canadian study plus concerns Amgen (the American company which owns the patent on the drug) have about safety, led Amgen to withdraw the GDNF product and halt all trials of its use. This move has caused much controversy since a number of patients receiving the drug on a trial basis were gaining substantial benefit from it. One such patient stated 'It was like getting my life back'. Some of the safety concerns are based on animal studies which showed that high doses of GDNF given to monkeys caused degenerative effects in the cerebellum, an area of the brain involved in the co-ordination of movement. However, data from studies carried out in patients with Parkinson's disease prior to the drug being withdrawn, showed no such problems.[26] Cerebellar tissue was evaluated in 59 animals that were treated with placebo or doses of GDNF that were higher than those used in the trials to treat Parkinson's disease. Cerebellar damage occurred in 4 out of the 15 monkeys given the highest dose of the drug. Postmortem studies carried out on the brain of a patient from Wales who had received the therapy, but died of an unrelated heart attack in 2005, showed that dopamine-containing nerve fibres lost in Parkinson's disease had sprouted back in the region where GDNF had been infused.[27] In other words, there was evidence his dopaminergic nerve fibres were regrowing. This finding has added to the frustration that further work with the drug has been halted. Although the evidence is based on very small numbers of patients, many people feel that GDNF really does offer an opportunity for producing dramatic results clinically, and the discovery at post mortem of nerve cell regrowth has added to the belief that this form of therapy should be pursued further. Steven Gill, neurosurgeon at the Frenchay Hospital in Bristol who carried out some of the trial work with GDNF, has stated that although the technique needs refining he believes this therapy might provide 'a chance to reverse the progress of Parkinson's' adding that it was potentially the most important step 'since the development of L-dopa'.[28] There is a growing lobby which is attempting to put pressure on Amgen to allow further research to take place with GDNF, but so far, the company has refused to supply the product for compassionate use.

For information on GDNF gene therapy see page 129.

Modulators of mitochondrial function

Creatine

A very pure form of creatine known as PD-02 has been assessed for its potential value in treating the symptoms of Parkinson's disease.[29] This was a Phase II study carried out in 200 patients at an early stage of their disease. Using the UPDRS, patients receiving PD-02 were found to have progressed more slowly after one year than those patients who received placebo. The results of animal studies suggest PD-02 has neuroprotective properties and might protect dopaminergic cells from damage caused by the condition. Clinical trials are at a very early stage, and these are needed to ascertain whether progression of Parkinson's disease can be slowed with this treatment.

Coenzyme Q₁₀

As discussed in Chapter 4, coenzyme Q_{10}, which is the electron acceptor for mitochondrial complex I and II, has been used for several years as a complementary therapy. Although the results of some studies have been encouraging,[30] further trials need to be carried out in order to assess its true value.

Growth factors

A constituent of brain cells known as GM1 is thought to stimulate growth factors, and in animal models of Parkinson's disease appears to have restorative and protective effects on dopamine cells.[31] When tried in patients with Parkinson's disease, some improvement in symptoms occurred and patients tolerated the GMI well, with no occurrence of serious adverse events.[32] A semi-synthetic derivative has now been produced called lysoganglioside which it is hoped will produce beneficial effects without the problems associated with GM1 administration.

Leteprinim is a small molecule which is able to cross the blood–brain barrier (growth factors themselves are too large). It mimics the effects of nerve growth factor and because of the size of the molecule can be administered orally or by injection and still be taken up by the brain. Once inside the brain, leteprinim activates the genes that are responsible for the production of growth factors. The results of animal studies are encouraging, but whether clinical benefits are achieved in humans remains to be seen.

Neuroimmunophilins

Much of the research effort to find ways of promoting neuroprotection and neurorestoration has focused on non-immunosuppressive immuno-philin ligands (NI-IPLs).[33] It is thought that NI-IPLs work through a variety of mechanisms which include activating effects on glutathione, neurotrophic factors, and possibly an anti-apoptic action. NI-IPLs do not cause side-effects associated with immune deficiency, since they do not have immunosuppressant properties.

Gene therapy

For some years, gene therapy has been highlighted as a potential break-through in the treatment of an ever-growing range of illnesses. The range includes Parkinson's disease and much research is taking place to see whether such therapy is indeed likely to halt or reverse the disease process. Gene therapy involves introducing specific genes into patients, either to take over the role of defective genes responsible for causing the condition, or to induce processes that prevent cell death or promote their regeneration. Genes which control the survival of dopamine-producing cells or increase the production of dopamine may successfully treat (or cure) Parkinson's disease if the appropriate areas of the brain can be targeted.

Ingenious mechanisms have been developed to 'carry' the gene material to the site where it is needed. Viruses that have been inactivated in terms of their ability to cause clinical infection can be used as gene carriers. Much work has been done with adenoviruses, into which are inserted the genes that encode for the desired factors to be produced. These factors may for example promote the survival and function of nerve cells (neurotrophic factors), or the regeneration of dopaminergic pathways (dopaminergic neuron differentiation factors). The virus containing the gene material which encodes for the relevant factors is injected into the appropriate part of the brain to ensure it targets the area where the encoding for the therapeutic compound is needed. A number of gene types are being studied for their potential to restore proper functioning of the pathways involved in Parkinson's disease. Some examples that may prove of value in Parkinson's disease are outlined below.

Growth factors

GDNF has been shown in animal models of Parkinson's disease to stimulate regrowth of cells.[34] Some recently published papers have also suggested this occurs in the human brain (see GDNF, page 127). Although GDNF can be injected directly into the brain, there are problems associated with this form of administration. An alternative is to use a virus to deliver the gene that encodes for the body's own production of this growth factor.

Glutamic acid decarboxylase

Excessive activity of glutamate receptors in the brain is thought to play a role in the occurrence of levodopa-induced dyskinesia. Progression of the disease may in part be caused by the increased damage and death of nerve cells resulting from the excessive glutamate activity. Glutamic acid decarboxylase (GAD) is a naturally occurring factor that deactivates glutamic acid and consequently prevents nerve cell damage. Material encoding for the production of GAD has been administered to humans using a virus as a carrier. It is too early to establish the effectiveness of this approach.

Dopaminergic neurons differentiation factors

Dopaminergic neurons differentiation factors (DNDF), including one known as 'sonic hedgehog' (named after the video game) are involved in the production of new dopamine cells in the brain of the fetus. The sonic hedgehog protein is involved in forming brain and other body tissue while in the womb. It is also found in areas of the adult brain involved in the control of movement. Although its specific role after birth is unknown, it has been suggested that it acts as a neurotransmitter controlling activity of the subthalamic nucleus. Animal work suggests sonic hedgehog may be reduced in Parkinson's disease. Further studies have shown that increasing the concentration of sonic hedgehog decreases the electrical activity in the subthalamic nucleus. In theory this could achieve the same effect as deep brain stimulation of the sub-thalamic nucleus (see page 98). The gene which produces sonic hedgehog has been isolated and inserted into a virus carrier. When delivered into the areas of brain laboratory animals, brain stem cells start dividing three times faster than normal and new neuron produc-tion is increased.[35] The use of gene therapy to promote this process is being further investigated.

Tyrosine hydroxylase

Tyrosine hydroxylase is crucial in the physiological production of dopamine within dopamine cells. Gene therapy can deliver the gene responsible for tyrosine hydroxylase production into the appropriate cells, leading to raised levels of dopamine.

Stem cells

Stem cells are the initial, undifferentiated cells from which specific cells specialising in particular roles are derived. If ways are found to steer stem cells into becoming particular type of cells, such as those producing dopamine, and these are implanted into the appropriate area of the body, it might be possible to replace or 'repair' deficiencies occurring because of disease. Stem cells which have been grown into dopamine-producing cells could be transplanted into the area of the brain where degeneration of the dopaminergic pathway has occurred, to re-establish neuronal circuits involved in controlling movement. Stem cell research to find a treatment for Parkinson's disease is focusing on the factors required to transform the undifferentiated cells into those that are required. Recent work has identified two transcription factor proteins, Lmx1a and Msx1. Expression of Lmx1a in embryonic stem cells resulted in the generation of dopamine neurons.[36] Furthermore, the dopamine neurons seem to be of the correct type found in the midbrain, increasing the chance that they will be suitable for replacing diseased or dead cells in Parkinson's disease.

The source of stem cells is derived from fetal tissue – for example from embryos created for *in vitro* fertilisation (IVF) but which are no longer needed. This technique has led to a great deal of controversy and raised a number of ethical and moral issues. In August 2006, scientists reported they had successfully developed a method of producing stem cells without destroying the embryos in the process. Single cells were removed from spare human IVF embryos. The embryos were left intact, which may reduce some of the controversy surrounding existing methods where the human embryo is destroyed.[37] However, many people will remain unhappy about the use of embryos as a laboratory tool believing this to be unethical even if the embryo is not damaged. Passionate arguments both for and against will persist until an alternative to using fetal tissue is found.

Tissue transplantation

The idea of transplanting tissue into areas of the brain where degeneration of neurons has occurred is not new. An enormous amount of effort has been put into research that endeavours to find ways of replacing or 'rebuilding' the dopaminergic pathways in the basal ganglia.

Adrenal gland tissue

As far back as the 1980s, tissue from one of the patient's own adrenal glands was used as a source for transplantation into the brain. Results from this technique have always been disappointing and is a strategy no longer used. More recently, attention has turned to other sources of tissue.

Human fetal tissue

Transplanted human fetal cells survive the transplantation process and have been shown to restore dopamine release in the striatum of patients with Parkinson's disease.[38] However, the clinical trials carried out so far indicate that little improvement occurs following the procedure. This is somewhat surprising since there are cases where significant benefit has been claimed in some patients receiving fetal tissue transplants.

Other sources of tissue

Various other sources of dopamine tissue are being tested for transplantation, including xenografts (tissue taken from one species and transplanted to another). Dopamine cells from pig embryos have been used, but as with the formal clinical trial using human tissue, no improvement in symptoms results. Cells from the patient's own carotid bodies may prove to be an effective source since these produce high levels of dopamine. Advances are being made in the implantation of other human tissue, for example, human retinal pigment epithelial cells (hRPE). An experimental product called Spheramine consists of hRPE cells attached to 'microcarriers' (microscopic gelatine beads). After implantation into the brain, the cells produce levodopa. Trials with this treatment are currently underway.

Non-invasive brain stimulation

Repetitive transcranial magnetic stimulation

This technique involves using repetitive transcranial magnetic stimulation (rTMS) over the supplementary motor area of the brain. It is hoped that in some way this can modify neuronal activity, leading to improvement in the symptoms of Parkinson's disease. A study has been carried out in a group of patients with advanced Parkinson's disease, the results of which suggest that drug-induced dyskinesias are markedly reduced.[39] The dyskinesias were induced by a continuous infusion of apomorphine. Experimenting with the frequency of the stimulation showed that rTMS at 1 Hz was much more effective than at 5 Hz. A meta-analysis of published trials has confirmed that rTMS has a significant effect on the motor function of patients with Parkinson's disease.[40] However, not all trials have produced a positive result, but this may be due to variations in the site of administration and other differences in technique, as well as differences in the duration of treatment. The mechanism for the therapeutic effect is not understood, but may be related to changes in the neuronal networks that connect with basal ganglia. One theory is that rTMS alters activity in cortical areas of the brain that are closely connected to the striatum and the subthalamic nucleus via glutamatergic pathways, which increases the release of dopamine in the basal ganglia. Alternatively, stimulation primarily directed towards cortical sites may compensate for abnormal activity in the cortex associated with Parkinson's disease. One study has assessed the effects of rTMS on depression associated with Parkinson's disease.[41] It was shown to be as effective as fluoxetine as measured on several rating scales. Adverse effects occurred more frequently in patients receiving fluoxetine.

Transcranial electric polarisation

Transcranial electric polarisation (TCEP) is a new idea developed at the Institute of Human Brain, Russian Academy of Sciences. The procedure involves placing electrodes on the scalp and passing a weak electrical current. Researchers claim that improvement is seen in patient's movement and inappropriate muscle tone is reduced.[42] It is also claimed that TCEP reduces the side-effects that patients experience from their drug therapy for Parkinson's disease. No improvement is seen in tremor. The procedure is carried out using 2 mA for 15 min three or four times a day on alternate days. TCEP is an interesting concept, but the value needs to be confirmed with properly conducted controlled studies.

Electroconvulsive therapy

A number of studies have been carried out to assess the value of electro-convulsive therapy (ECT) in the treatment of Parkinson's disease. The procedure involves giving a strong pulse of electrical current through an electrode placed on the head to induce a seizure. Although the mechanism by which ECT produces its effects is not known, it has been used as a successful treatment of severe depression for many years. A meta-analysis has been carried out of published studies to determine the effectiveness of ECT in treating the motor symptoms of Parkinson's disease.[40] Although limited by the low number of trials that meet the criteria for inclusion in the meta-analysis, the outcome did suggest that ECT can be effective. Further well-designed trials are needed to clearly establish what role ECT may have in the clinical management of patients with Parkinson's disease.

Diagnostic developments

A molecular-imaging agent has been developed which specifically binds to the dopamine transporter protein present on the surface of dopamine-producing neurons. This protein is produced exclusively by dopamine-containing cells in the brain. Using single photon emission computed tomography (SPECT) imaging, it is possible to visualise these neurons and assess whether they are present in normal amounts. The highly selective imaging agent called Altropane could help in the diagnosis of Parkinson's disease, since in this condition the SPECT image would show a decrease in dopaminergic neurons, whereas in other conditions with similar symptoms the density of dopamine cells would look normal. Studies of misdiagnosis rates, especially in the early stages of the disease, vary, but are quite high. Altropane may become a valuable aid in differentiating between parkinsonian and non-parkinsonian tremors. This is important clinically, since the appropriate management of the two conditions is different. A Phase III study of the agent is under way to assess its use and reliability.

References

1. Katzenschlager R, Evans A, Manson A, *et al*. *Mucuna pruriens* in Parkinson's disease: a double blind clinical and pharmacological study. *J Neurol Neurosurg Psychiatry* 2004; 75: 1672–1677.
2. Blindauer KA. A randomised controlled trial of etilevodopa in patients with Parkinson's disease who have motor fluctuations. *Arch Neurol* 2006; 63: 210–216.
3. Clarke CE, Guttman M. Dopamine agonist monotherapy in Parkinson's disease. *Lancet* 2002; 360: 1767–1769.
4. Frachiewicz EJ, Jhee SS, Shiovitz TM, *et al*. Brasofensine treatment for Parkinson's disease in combination with levodopa/carbidopa. *Ann Pharmacother* 2002; 36: 225–230.
5. Murata M, Horiuchi E, Kanazawa I. Zonisamide has beneficial effects on Parkinson's disease patients. *Neurosci Res* 2001; 41: 397–399.
6. Murata M, Hasegawa K, Kanazawa I. Zonisamide improves motor function in Parkinson's disease: a randomised, double-blind study. *Neurology* 2007; 68: 45–50.
7. Savola JM, Hill M, Engstrom M, *et al*. Fipamezole (JP-1730) is a potent alpha2 adrenergic receptor antagonist that reduces levodopa-induced dyskinesia in the MPTP-lesioned primate model of Parkinson's disease. *Mov Disord* 2003; 18: 872–883.
8. Oy Juvantia Pharma Ltd. Press release 28 June 2004. *Juvantia Pharma Announces Positive Results of Phase IIa study in Parkinson's Disease*. Results presented at Movement Disorder Society's 8th International Congress of Parkinson's Disease and Movement Disorders in Rome, Italy, 2004.

www.biofund.fi/images/PR_ENG_FIPAMEZOLE_28.6.2004.pdf (accessed 17 July 2007).

9. Kanda T, Jackson MJ, Smith LA, et al. Combined use of the adenosine A(2A) antagonist KW-6002 with L-DOPA or with selective D1 or D2 dopamine agonists increases antiparkinsonian activity but not dyskinesia in MPTP-treated monkeys. *Exp Neurol* 2000; 162: 321–327.

10. Pinna A, Wardas J, Simola N, Morelli M. New therapies for the treatment of Parkinson's disease: adenosine A2A receptor antagonists. *Life Sci* 2005; 12: 3259–3267.

11. Hauser RA, Hubble JO, Truong DD, et al. Randomised trial of the adenosine A2A receptor antagonist istradefylline in advanced Parkinson's disease. *Neurology* 2003; 61: 297–303.

12. Gillard M, Chatelain P, Fuks B. Binding characteristics of levetiracetam to synaptic vesicle protein 2A (SV2A) in human brain and in CHO cells expressing the human recombinant protein. *Eur J Pharmacol* 2006; 536: 102–108.

13. Loscher W, Honack D, Bloms-Funke P. The novel antiepileptic drug levetiracetam (ucb L059) induces alterations in GABA metabolism and turnover in discrete areas of rat brain and reduces neuronal activity in substantia nigra pars reticulata. *Brain Res* 1996; 735: 208–216.

14. Zesiewicz TA, Sullivan KL, Maldonado JL, et al. Open-label pilot study of levetiracetam (Keppra) for the treatment of levodopa-induced dyskinesias in Parkinson's disease. *Mov Disord* 2005; 20: 1205–1209.

15. Bara-Jimenez W, Bibbiani F, Morris MJ, et al. Effects of serotonin 5-HT1A agonist in advanced Parkinson's disease. *Mov Disord* 2005; 20: 932–936.

16. Venderova K, Ruzicka E, Vorisek V, Visnovsky P. Survey on cannabis use in Parkinson's disease: subjective improvement in motor symptoms. *Mov Disord* 2004; 19: 1102–1106.

17. Muller-Vahl KR, Kolbe H, Schneider U, Emrich HM. Cannabis in movement disorders. *Forsch Komplementarmed* 1999; 6 (Suppl 3): 23–27.

18. Caroll CB, Bain PG, Teare L, et al. Cannabis for dyskinesia in Parkinson's disease: a randomized double-blind crossover study. *Neurology* 2004; 63: 1245–1250.

19. Jankovic J, Hunter C. A double-blind, placebo-controlled and longitudinal study of riluzole in early Parkinson's disease. *Parkinsonism Relat Disord* 2002; 8: 271–276.

20. Koller W, Olanow CW, Rodnitzky R, et al. Effects of tocopherol and deprenyl on the progression of disability in early Parkinson's disease. *N Engl J Med* 1993; 328: 176–183.

21. Schapira AHV, Olanow CW. Neuroprotection in Parkinson disease: mysteries, myths, and misconceptions. *JAMA* 2004; 291: 358–364.

22. Boll JB, Geist MA, Kaminski-Schierle GS, et al. Improvement of embryonic dopaminergic neurone survival in culture and after grafting into the striatum of hemiparkinsonian rats by CEP-1347. *J Neurochem* 2004; 88: 698–707.

23. Patel NK, Bunnage M, Plaha P, et al. Intraputamenal infusion of glial cell line-derived neurotrophic factor in PD: a two-year outcome study. *Ann Neurol* 2005; 57: 298–302.

24. Slevin JT, Gerhardt GA, Smith CD, et al. Improvement of bilateral motor

functions in patients with Parkinson disease through the unilateral intra-putaminal infusion of glial cell line-derived neurotrophic factor. *J Neurosurg* 2005; 102: 216–222.

25. Lang AE, Gill S, Patel NK, *et al.* Randomized controlled trial of intra-putamenal glial cell line-derived neurotrophic factor infusion in Parkinson disease. *Ann Neurol* 2006; 59: 459–466.

26. Hooper R. Parkinson's drug prompts brain cell growth. *NewScientist.com News Service* 1 July 2005. www.newscientist.com/article.ns?id=dn7619 (accessed 17 July 2007).

27. Love S, Plaha P, Patel NK, *et al.* Glial cell line-derived neurotrophic factor induces neuronal sprouting in human brain. *Nat Med* 2005; 11: 703.

28. Parkinson's drug 'highly promising'. *BBC News* 31 March 2003. http://news.bbc.co.uk/1/hi/health/2892283.stm (accessed 17 July 2007).

29. The NINDS NET-PD Investigators. A randomised, double-blind, futility clinical trial of creatine and minocycline in early Parkinson's disease. *Neurology* 2006; 66: 664–671.

30. Muller T, Buttner T, Gholipour AF, *et al.* Coenzyme Q10 supplementation provides mild symptomatic benefit in patients with Parkinson's disease. *Neurosci Lett* 2003; 341: 201–204.

31. Goettl VM, Wemlinger TA, Duchemin AM, *et al.* GM1 ganglioside restores dopaminergic neurochemical and morphological markers in aged rats. *Neuroscience* 1999; 92: 991–1000.

32. Schneider JS, Roeltgen DP, Mancall EL, *et al.* Parkinson's disease: improved function with GM1 ganglioside treatment in a randomized placebo-controlled study. Neurology 1998; 50: 1630–1636.

33. Tanaka K, Ogawa N. Possibility of non-immunosuppressive immunophilin ligands as potential therapeutic agents in Parkinson's disease. *Curr Pharm Design* 2004; 10: 669–677.

34. Grondin R, Zhang Z, Yi A, *et al.* Chronic, controlled GDNF infusion promotes structural and functional recovery in advanced parkinsonian monkeys. *Brain* 2002; 125: 2191–2201.

35. Torres EM, Monville C, Lowenstein PR, *et al.* Delivery of sonic hedgehog or glial cell derived neurotrophic factor to dopamine-rich grafts in a rat model of Parkinson's disease using adenoviral vectors – increased yield of dopamine cells is dependent on embryonic donor age. *Brain Res Bull* 2005; 68: 31–41.

36. Andersson E, Tryggvason U, Deng Q, *et al.* Identification of intrinsic determinants of midbrain dopamine neurons. *Cell* 2006; 124: 393–405.

37. Pearson H. Early embryos can yield stem cells and survive. *Nature* 2006; 442: 858.

38. Lindvall O, Hagell P. Cell therapy and transplantation in Parkinson's disease. *Clin Chem Lab Med* 2001; 39: 356–361.

39. Koch G, Brusa L, Caltagirone C, *et al.* rTMS of supplementary motor area modulates therapy-induced dyskinesias in Parkinson's disease. *Neurology* 2005; 65: 623–625.

40. Fregni F, Simon DK, Wu A, Pacual-Leone A. Non-invasive brain stimulation for Parkinson's disease: a systematic review and meta-analysis of the literature. *J Neurol Neurosurg Psychiatry* 2005; 76: 1614–1623.

41. Fregni F, Santos CM, Myczkowski ML, *et al.* Repetitive transcranial magnetic

stimulation is as effective as fluoxetine in the treatment of depression in patients with Parkinson's disease. *J Neurol Neurosurg Psychiatry* 2004; 75: 1171–1174.

42. Parkinson's disease may be treated by electric current. *Medical News Today* March 2006. www.medicalnewstoday.com/medicalnews.php?newsid=40260 (accessed 17 July 2007).

Further reading

Chan KL, Jagait P, Tugwell C. Parkinson's disease – current and future aspects of drug treatment. *Hosp Pharm* 2004; 11: 18–22.

Clarke CE. A 'cure' for Parkinson's disease: can neuroprotection be proven with current trial designs? *Mov Disord* 2004; 19: 491–499.

Clarke CE. Neuroprotection and pharmacotherapy for motor symptoms in Parkinson's disease. *Lancet Neurol* 2004; 3: 466–475.

Johnston TH, Brotchie JM. Drugs in development for Parkinson's disease: an update. *Curr Opin Investig Drugs* 2006; 7: 25–32.

Koller WC, Tse W. Unmet medical needs in Parkinson's disease. *Neurology* 2004; 62 (1 Suppl 1): S1–8.

Kuan WL, Barker RA. New therapeutic approaches to Parkinson's disease including neural transplants. *Neurorehabil Neural Repair* 2005; 19: 155–181.

Ravina BM, Fagan SC, Hart RG. Neuroprotective agents for clinical trials in Parkinson's disease. *Neurology* 2003; 60: 1234–1240.

Shapira AH. Present and future drug treatment for Parkinson's disease. *J Neurol Neurosurg Psychiatry* 2005; 76: 1472–1478.

8

Patient care and service provision

The National Service Framework for Long Term Conditions[1]

Quality requirement 2 of *The National Service Framework for Long Term Conditions* covers the early recognition, prompt diagnosis and treatment. The prime aim is to ensure that people presenting with neurological symptoms or a neurological condition receive the correct diagnosis and appropriate treatment as soon as possible. The National Service Framework (NSF) sets as a requirement that people suspected of having a neurological condition are to have prompt access to specialist neurological expertise for an accurate diagnosis and treatment as close to home as possible.

Recognition and diagnosis

The NSF recognises that people with long-term neurological conditions have improved health outcomes and better quality of life when they are able to access prompt specialist expertise to obtain a diagnosis and begin treatment. *The NHS Improvement Plan: putting people at the heart of public services* and *National Standards, Local Action: Health and Social Care Standards and Planning Framework 2005/6–2007/8* state that, by December 2008, no one should wait longer than 18 weeks from general practitioner (GP) referral to hospital treatment.[2,3]

Each year around one person in ten consults their GP about a neurological symptom. However, the document acknowledges that their first point of contact may be other healthcare professionals in the community, such as pharmacists.

It is important that people who may have a long-term neurological condition have a specialist assessment, since some diseases can be difficult to identify as they lack clear, simple diagnostic features. Parkinson's disease is an example – many patients with early stages of the disease having been wrongly diagnosed with arthritis, stroke, or considered to be suffering from the unfortunate but normal process of ageing.

The NSF outlines a number of steps that could be taken to improve the diagnosis of neurological conditions such as Parkinson's disease:

- primary care teams collaborating more closely with their linked neurologists
- improved training in recognising important symptoms for all staff likely to have contact with people first presenting with neurological problems
- triage of patients so that clinicians with the most appropriate skills, including practitioners with a special interest, evaluate people
- agreed protocols for timely referral for specialist neurological assessment and diagnostic tests as appropriate, which allow tests to be pre-booked and avoid unnecessary duplication of tests
- specialist clinics (e.g. in primary care settings) as close to people's homes as possible.

Treatment

The NSF emphasises the need for newly diagnosed patients to gain access to the full range of treatment and support services that may be necessary. It also states that they should be provided with information about treatment options, their effectiveness and any potential problems and side-effects, so they can make informed choices.

The effective use of medicines is often a fundamental aspect of the overall management of neurological conditions. It is concerning that research has shown that around 50% of medicines for long-term conditions are not taken as prescribed. People's beliefs and preferences about medicines are major factors in deciding if, and how, they use them. The NSF highlights a number of issues that are particularly relevant to Parkinson's disease and epilepsy, and states that in addition to providing information, it is essential that healthcare professionals:

- discuss the person's views and preferences with them
- reach a shared agreement about the proposed form of treatment
- make sure that people have the physical and cognitive skills to manage their medication themselves, or that there are appropriate arrangements to ensure that people take their medicines correctly
- provide contact details so that the person can get in touch straight away if they experience any problems with their medicines
- contact the person soon after treatment is started to ensure that there are no problems in taking their medicine.

The occurrence of side-effects with drug therapy for Parkinson's disease is common, and the NSF clearly indicates that patients may need advice and support in managing side-effects or, if they are considering stopping treatment, should have the opportunity to discuss this. Regular reviews of medication are important, especially for patients taking three or more medicines. The NSF states these should be carried out by 'a skilled reviewer (e.g. an appropriately trained pharmacist)'. This is to assess how they are taking their medicines, whether they are tolerating them, and the impact (both positive and negative) of medicines on their condition and on other aspects of their lives. The reviewer can agree adjustment of medication with the patient.

Quality requirement 11 of *The National Service Framework for Long Term Conditions* covers caring for people with neurological conditions in hospital or other health and social care settings. The aim of this requirement is to provide people suffering from long-term neurological conditions with appropriate neurological care at all times while they are having treatment or care in any health or social care setting. Their needs should continue to be met even if they are receiving care for other reasons.

When a person is admitted to hospital or another unfamiliar care setting (e.g. for an unrelated illness or for respite care), it is important that their normal neurological care plan continues as far as possible, for example:

- people with Parkinson's disease need their medication at specific times to control their symptoms properly. Failure to achieve this can result in poorer control of their symptoms and further medical problems developing
- people who normally self-medicate will need help to continue to do so while in hospital or other care settings if they are able to
- some people with long-term neurological conditions may need specialist aids and equipment (e.g. communication aids, equipment for feeding, walking aids, or specialist wheelchairs) to help them continue to function effectively during their stay in a hospital or care facility
- people who have cognitive and/or communication problems have particular needs of which staff may have little experience.

In the case of planned admissions, making the person's neurological care plan (which might include information on current medication, care programme and handling procedures) available to all staff so that appropriate arrangements can be made before the admission, will help ensure that the patient's neurological needs can be met. People with long-term neurological conditions who need treatment for other unrelated conditions, need to know how their neurological needs will be met in the non-specialist setting. Failure to provide this information can be a great source of anxiety for patients. It is also important that they are offered the opportunity to discuss any implications of their treatment on their neurological condition.

To help maintain high-quality care for people whenever they are in a non-neurological setting (e.g. a general hospital ward or care facility), good practice will ensure:

- an integrated neurological care plan is available to all staff
- there is close liaison with the patient's usual neurological care team
- in the case of planned admission, a pre-admission interview establishes any special needs, including for equipment provision, communication aids and transport
- there is effective consultation with the person about their management and, where appropriate, involvement of family/carers who are familiar with the person's care
- specialist advice and training for staff in general hospital and other care settings is available as necessary.

Chapter 4 of the NSF is entitled 'National support for local action' and signposts initiatives that can support local delivery of the NSF. It is broken down into several sections which are outlined below. Several of these are relevant and applicable to the management of Parkinson's disease and the provision of services to these patients.

National modernisation programmes

Action on Neurology

The Department of Health has been working with the NHS Modernisation Agency on the Action on Neurology programme to develop new ways of working to improve access and quality of care for people with neurological conditions. The outcomes of the programme will be available in their final report[4] (see www.modern.nhs.uk/action-on).

Neuroscience Critical Care Report

The Modernisation Agency published the *Neuroscience Critical Care Report – Progress in Developing Services* (August 2004) as part of its Critical Care Programme.[5]

National underpinning programmes

Finance

Extra resources for the NHS were announced in the 2003 Budget. As a result, the Department of Health was able to announce revenue allocations for 2003/2006 of £148 billion to primary care trusts (PCTs) over 3 years – a total cash increase of 30.83%. This gave PCTs 3 years of certainty of funding for the first time. In February 2005, the Department of Health announced a further £135 billion for the next two years 2006/2007 and 2007/2008 – a cash increase of 19.5%. This will again give PCTs certainty of funding for the next 3 years. In addition, as part of the recently announced Local Government Finance Settlement, the Department of Health notified local authorities of £11 448 million of revenue funding for adult personal social services (PSS) for 2005/2006. This reflects an 8% increase in the total funds (revenue and capital) allocated for adult PSS when compared with 2004/2005 unadjusted figures. PSS allocations are currently made to local authorities on an annual basis.

Workforce

In planning and delivering neurological and community services, it is important that there are enough staff with the right skills and experience who are well led, supported and deliver high-quality care. The Department of Health has established the Long Term Conditions Care Group Workforce Team (LTC CGWT), which is taking a national view on the health and social care workforce pressures of this NSF. The responsibility for supporting the CGWTs has been transferred to Skills for Health, which is also developing a competency framework on behalf of the LTC CGWT, defining the skills and knowledge needed to deliver the NSF. It will support service redesign and assessment of skill mix.[6]

The nursing profession

Several initiatives highlight the contribution of nurses to support the delivery of this NSF, including:

- *Making a Difference. Strengthening the nursing, midwifery and health visiting contribution to health and healthcare* (1999)[7]
- *The Chief Nursing Officer's 10 Key Roles for Nursing* (1999).[8] The *NHS Plan* requires NHS employers to empower appropriately qualified nurses, midwives and therapists to undertake a wider range of clinical tasks[9]

- *Liberating the Talents* describes continuing care, rehabilitation, managing long-term conditions and delivering the NSFs as core functions for all nurses in primary and community care[10]
- nurse prescribing, including:
  - independent prescribing for nursing[11]
  - supplementary prescribing[12]
  - patient group directions[13]
- case management/community matrons. *The NHS Improvement Plan: putting people at the heart of public services* (2004) sets out the government's intention that by 2008 there will be 3000 community matrons using case management techniques for planning and co-ordinating the care of people with high-intensity needs.[2] Community matrons will be key to delivering the Public Service Agreement target for long-term conditions.

Allied health professions

A number of initiatives highlight the contribution that allied health professions (AHPs) can make to support the delivery of this NSF, including:

- *Meeting the Challenge: a strategy for the allied health professions* (2000)[14] illustrates how the role of AHPs can be developed and supported and the central role they have to play in delivering the *NHS Plan*[9] and *NHS Improvement Plan*[2]
- *The Chief Health Professions Officer's 10 Key Roles for AHPs* (2003) describes the current roles of AHPs and examines the potential for new roles to be developed[15]
- extending non-medical prescribing to a range of healthcare professionals including AHPs[16]
- *The National Primary and Care Trust (NatPaCT) Self-Assessment Tool for AHPs* (2003) highlights significant issues for the delivery, modernisation and commissioning of AHP services.[17]

Pharmacy profession and medicines management

Several initiatives have been developed that will increase the contribution that pharmacy can make to support the delivery of this NSF:

- *A Vision for Pharmacy in the New NHS* (July 2003) emphasises the contribution of pharmacy to high-quality, person-centred NHS services in community pharmacies, other primary care settings and hospitals.[18]

- *The Chief Pharmaceutical Officer's 10 Key Roles* (July 2003) focuses on the role of the pharmacy profession in providing high-quality services to people[18]
- *Extending prescribing: a framework* is being developed for independent prescribing by pharmacists, in particular for people with long-term conditions[19]
- the new contractual framework for community pharmacy, will provide services such as repeat dispensing, medicine usage review, signposting and support for self-care[20]
- the medicines management collaborative, which is hosted by the National Prescribing Centre, provides medicines management schemes to help people get the most from their medicines. The collaborative programme currently covers 146 PCTs, involving around 14 000 GPs and 4900 community pharmacies. It has the potential to ensure over 27 million people across these PCTs can get help to make better use of their medicines.[21]

Medicines management

The Department of Health has published *Management of Medicines: a resource to support implementation of the wider aspects of medicines management for the National Service Frameworks for Diabetes, Renal Services and Long-term Conditions* (July 2004). It offers practical support for PCTs and NHS trusts.[22]

Medicines partnership

The Department of Health is funding the Medicines Partnership based at the Royal Pharmaceutical Society.

It has developed two guides to help people prepare for review consultations: (see www.medicinespartnership.org/medicationreview/focusonyourmedicines):

- *Focus on your Medicines,*[23] which is suitable for all conditions
- *Focus on your Health for People with Epilepsy,*[24] which includes an epilepsy diary for the person to complete and questions to consider.

The Medicines Partnership also offers an interactive website to help people with multiple sclerosis who are considering disease-modifying drugs make an informed decision about treatment options.[25]

The Medicines Partnership is also running a major study to develop community pharmacists with a special interest in Parkinson's disease who can support people to understand and manage their medicines. The project aims to lead to a framework for pharmacists with a special interest in specific neurological conditions.[26]

Medicines information project

The Medicines Partnership, NHS Direct Online, the Medicines and Healthcare Products Regulatory Agency (MHRA) and the pharmaceutical industry are collaborating on a new, independent, comprehensive source of medicines information for people, linked to information about conditions and treatment options. They have already developed a complete set of 'medicines guides' for epilepsy. Further conditions will be added over the next 2–3 years. The guides are available through NHS Direct Online.[27]

Practitioners with a special interest (PwSI)

Practitioners with special interests (PwSIs), including GPs (GPwSI), nurses (NwSI) and AHPs (AHPwSI) and, in future, pharmacists, make it possible to provide a wide range of services in local community settings. The PwSI approach is being extended with further frameworks for healthcare scientists and other key staff.[28] NatPaCT has also produced documentation and support on PwSIs.[29]

Research and development

The Department of Health has funded short-term research studies focusing on user/carer experience and sudden brain injury to support the development of the NSF. There is funding for a longer-term, more intensive programme of research to support implementation of the NSF and examine its impact on the management of long-term neurological conditions.

NSF for Long-term Conditions Information Strategy

The NSF Information Strategy is a web-based resource for use alongside the NSF. It is designed to signpost tools, evidence and other sources of information that will help implement and deliver the NSF.[30]

Parkinson's Disease – National Clinical Guideline for the Diagnosis and Management in Primary and Secondary Care

In the summer of 2006, the National Institute for Health and Clinical Excellence (NICE) published guidelines for the diagnosis and management of Parkinson's disease in primary and secondary care.[31] The work was carried out by a Guideline Development Group set up by the National Collaborating Centre for Chronic Conditions. A much larger document was published by the Royal College of Physicians,[32] which includes details of how the recommendations were developed, and summarises the evidence on which they were based. Funded and produced for the NHS by NICE, the review has been based on the best evidence that could be found in the published literature; in excess of 400 references are quoted in the document.

Two further publications have been produced: a quick reference guide intended for healthcare professionals,[33] and a separate document information for people with Parkinson's disease and their carers.[34] All of these can be downloaded from the NICE website.

The NICE guideline,[31] which aims to set out best practice for the diagnosis and management of Parkinson's disease, covers the following areas:

- diagnosis and monitoring
- communication and education
- pharmacotherapy (prevention of progression)
- pharmacotherapy (functional disability in early disease)
- adjuvant pharmacotherapy (functional disability in late disease)
- non-pharmacological management
- neuropsychiatric conditions
- palliative care.

It does not cover therapies such as fetal cell transplantation; stem cells; gene therapy; drugs that block the action of glutamate; glial cell-derived neurotrophic factor (GDNF); and viral transfection, although most of these potential forms of treatment are discussed elsewhere in this book (see Chapter 7).

In assessing the performance of the NHS, the Healthcare Commission will be using the clinical guideline to establish whether standards have been met. Therefore, its content should be taken into account by NHS organisations when planning and delivering care.

A number of recommendations are made on areas that need further research. These include: neuroprotection in an attempt to find a 'cure' for the disease; the use of agents to treat dementia and depression associated with Parkinson's disease; the role of supportive therapies such as physiotherapy, occupational therapy and speech and language therapy; and further work on which diagnostic investigations for Parkinson's disease and potential biomarkers of its progression are clinically useful and cost-effective.

The NICE guideline makes a large number of recommendations with a view to improving the quality of care given to patients suffering with Parkinson's disease.[31] These span a range of aspects including the communication needs of patients and their carers, the diagnosis of Parkinson's disease, and the pharmacological treatment of the symptoms of the condition. Recommendations are also made on the non-motor features of the disease, the use of surgery and other interventions, and palliative care.

The following section provides an overview of the recommendation made within each of the key sections of the document.

Overview of recommendations made in the national guideline

Communication with people with Parkinson's disease and their carers

- Whenever communicating with people who have Parkinson's disease, the aim should be towards empowering them to participate in the judgements and choices regarding their own care (Recommendation 1).
- Discussions should be aimed at achieving a balance between the provision of honest, realistic information about the condition and promoting a feeling of optimism (Recommendation 2).
- Since people with Parkinson's disease may develop impaired cognitive ability, a communication deficit and/or depression, they should be provided with:
  - both oral and written communication throughout the course of the disease, which should be individually tailored and reinforced as necessary
  - consistent communication from the various professionals involved (Recommendation 3).
- Families and carers should be given information about the condition, their entitlements to care assessment and the range of support services available (Recommendation 4).
- People with Parkinson's disease should have a comprehensive care plan agreed between themselves, their family and/or carers and specialist and secondary healthcare providers (Recommendation 5).

- People with Parkinson's disease should be offered an accessible point of contact with relevant specialist services. This could be provided by a Parkinson's disease nurse specialist (Recommendation 6).
- All people with Parkinson's disease who drive should be advised to inform the Driver and Vehicle Licensing Agency (DVLA) and their car insurer of their condition at the time of diagnosis (Recommendation 7) (see also Appendix D).

Diagnosing Parkinson's disease

- Parkinson's disease should be considered as a possible diagnosis in patients who present with tremor, stiffness, slowness, balance problems and/or gait disorders (Recommendation 8).
- The UK Parkinson's Disease Society Brain Bank Criteria should be used as the basis for making a clinical diagnosis of Parkinson's disease (see Box 2.2, page 25) (Recommendation 9).
- Clinicians are encouraged to discuss with patients their feelings about tissue donation to a brain bank since this may be valuable in confirming the diagnosis, as well as furthering research (Recommendation 10).
- If a patient is suspected of having Parkinson's disease, they should be referred quickly and untreated to a specialist with expertise in the differential diagnosis of this condition. If the symptoms are mild, the patient should be seen within 6 weeks, but new referrals in later disease with more complex problems should be seen within 2 weeks (Recommendation 11).
- Patients with a diagnosis of Parkinson's disease should be seen at regular intervals of between 6 and 12 months in order to review their diagnosis. The diagnosis should be reconsidered if atypical clinical features develop (Recommendation 12).
- Single photon emission computed tomography (SPECT) is considered to have limited use. However, it can be useful in people with tremor where essential tremor cannot be clinically differentiated from parkinsonism (Recommendation 13).
- 123I-FP-CIT SPECT should be available to specialists with expertise in its use and interpretation (Recommendation 14).
- Positron emission tomography (PET) should not be used in the differential diagnosis of parkinsonian syndromes, except in the context of clinical trials (Recommendation 15).
- Although in expert hands structural magnetic resonance imaging (MRI) has proved to be of some value in differentiating Parkinson's disease from other types of parkinsonism, there is insufficient evidence for it to be

recommended in the differential diagnosis of Parkinson's disease (Recommendation 16).

- Structural MRI may be considered for the differential diagnosis of parkinsonian syndromes (Recommendation 17).
- Magnetic resonance volumetry should not be used in the differential diagnosis of parkinsonian syndromes, except in the context of clinical trials. Further work showing its value is required before it can be recommended (Recommendation 18).
- Magnetic resonance spectroscopy (MRS) has produced contradictory results in terms of its value; it is therefore recommended that it is not used in the differential diagnosis of parkinsonian syndromes (Recommendation 19).
- Acute levodopa and apomorphine challenge tests should not be used in the differential diagnosis of parkinsonian syndromes. It is considered they add nothing to standard chronic levodopa therapy in the differentiation of established cases of Parkinson's disease from other causes of parkinsonism. However, the acute apomorphine challenge test may be useful in assessing whether a person with later Parkinson's disease will still respond to dopaminergic drug therapy (Recommendation 20).
- Objective smell testing is not recommended for use in the differential diagnosis of parkinsonian syndromes, except in the context of clinical trials. There is currently little evidence that objective smell testing is able to differentiate Parkinson's disease from other parkinsonian syndromes (Recommendation 21).

Neuroprotection

- Vitamin E has not been shown to be neuroprotective in Parkinson's disease and is therefore not recommended (Recommendation 22).
- Coenzyme Q_{10} has produced encouraging results in some trials, though most of these are small. Until further evidence is available, coenzyme Q_{10} should not be used as a neuroprotective therapy for people with Parkinson's disease except in the context of clinical trials (Recommendation 23).
- Dopamine agonists such as ropinirole and pramipexole have, in some studies, shown they may have neuroprotective properties. However, the methodology of these studies has been criticised and mechanisms other than neuroprotection may be responsible for any delay in the development of motor symptoms that has been observed. It is therefore recommended that dopamine agonists should not be used as neuroprotective therapies for people with Parkinson's disease except in the context of clinical trials (Recommendation 24).
- Monoamine oxidase type-B (MAO-B) inhibitors (selegiline and rasagiline)

may have anti-apoptotic effects. However, long-term follow-up studies of sufficient size are required to assess whether the MAO-B inhibitors have neuroprotective properties in Parkinson's disease. It is therefore recommended that they should not be used as neuroprotective therapies for people with Parkinson's disease except in the context of clinical trials (Recommendation 25).

Symptomatic pharmacological therapy in Parkinson's disease

Early pharmacological therapy

- The large ELLDOPA trial has confirmed that levodopa is the most effective treatment for Parkinson's disease and therefore it is recommended that this drug may be used as a symptomatic treatment for people with early Parkinson's disease (Recommendation 26).

- The dose of levodopa should be kept as low as possible in order to maintain good function and reduce the development of motor complications (Recommendation 27).

- Dopamine agonists may be used for the symptomatic treatment of early Parkinson's disease (Recommendation 28).

- The dose of dopamine agonist should be titrated until a clinically useful effect is attained. If side-effects prevent this, another agonist (or a drug from another class) should be used instead (Recommendation 29).

- Since ergot-derived dopamine agonists have the potential to produce serious toxic effects, patients receiving these drugs should have, as a minimum, renal function tests, erythrocyte sedimentation rate (ESR) and chest radiograph before starting treatment, and every year thereafter (Recommendation 30).

- Non-ergot-derived agonists are preferred in most cases due to the monitoring which is necessary with ergot-derived dopamine agonists (Recommendation 31).

- MAO-B inhibitors have been shown to improve motor symptoms, improve activities of daily living and delay the need for levodopa. They may therefore be used as a symptomatic treatment for people with early Parkinson's disease (Recommendation 32).

- There is limited evidence for the efficacy or safety of beta-adrenergic antagonists in Parkinson's disease, however these drugs may be used for the symptomatic treatment of selected people with postural tremor associated with Parkinson's disease, but should not be regarded as drugs of first choice (Recommendation 33).

- Amantadine may be used as a treatment for people with early Parkinson's disease, but should not be regarded as a drug of first choice. There is less evidence available on its efficacy and safety compared to other drugs such as levodopa and dopamine agonists, and therefore these are considered more appropriate treatments for the early stages of the disease (Recommendation 34).

- Anticholinergic drugs often cause neuropsychiatric side-effects and data are limited on the efficacy of these drugs in the treatment of Parkinson's disease. However, they may be used as a symptomatic treatment (typically in young people) with early Parkinson's disease and severe tremor, providing the patient has no cognitive dysfunction. If used, treatment should be regularly reviewed. Withdrawal can sometimes be difficult due to the re-emergence of motor impairments (Recommendation 35).

- Available evidence suggests that modified-release levodopa preparations are not beneficial in delaying the onset of motor complications in people with early Parkinson's disease (Recommendation 36).

- It is considered that there is no single drug of first choice for people with early Parkinson's disease. It is hoped the UK PD MED trial (using quality-of-life and health economics outcome measures) will show any differences there may be between levodopa, dopamine agonists and MAO-B inhibitors, but at present it is not possible to identify a universal first-choice drug therapy. Therefore, the choice of drug first prescribed should take into account the following:
  - clinical and lifestyle characteristics
  - patient preference, after the patient has been informed of the short-term and long-term benefits and drawbacks of the drug classes (Recommendation 37).

Later pharmacological therapy

- There is some evidence that modified-release levodopa preparations can reduce motor fluctuations. However, doubts have been expressed on the validity of the results from these trials. Therefore it is recommended that modified-release levodopa preparations may be used to reduce motor complications in people with later Parkinson's disease but should not be regarded as drugs of first choice (Recommendation 38).

- Dopamine agonists may be used to reduce motor fluctuations in people with later Parkinson's disease (Recommendation 39).

- If an ergot-derived dopamine agonist is used, it is important the patient has, as a minimum, renal function tests, ESR and chest radiograph performed before starting treatment and each year thereafter (Recommendation 40).

- The dosage of dopamine agonist should be titrated until a clinically useful effect is achieved. If side-effects prevent this, then another drug should be used instead (Recommendation 41).

- Non-ergot-derived agonists are preferred in most cases due to the monitoring which is necessary with ergot-derived dopamine agonists (Recommendation 42).
- MAO-B inhibitors may be used to reduce motor fluctuations in people with later Parkinson's disease, although evidence for their long-term benefits is limited (Recommendation 43).
- Since catechol-O-methyl transferase inhibitors reduce 'off-time' and allow a reduction in levodopa dose, while improving 'on-time', motor impairments and disability, they may be used to reduce motor fluctuations in people with later Parkinson's disease (Recommendation 44).
- In view of problems with reduced concordance, people with later Parkinson's disease taking entacapone should be offered a triple combination preparation of levodopa, carbidopa and entacapone (Stalevo) (Recommendation 45).
- Since tolcapone has caused rare cases of fatal hepatic toxicity and neuroleptic malignant syndrome, its use in England and Wales is limited to patients with later Parkinson's disease who have failed on entacapone due to lack of efficacy or side-effects. Liver function tests need to be carried out every 2 weeks during the first year of therapy, and thereafter in accordance with the summary of product characteristics (Recommendation 46).
- Amantadine may be used to reduce dyskinesia in people with later Parkinson's disease, although data on its long-term effects are lacking. Evidence from one trial suggests the anti-dyskinetic effect of the drug is substantially reduced after 8 months of therapy (Recommendation 47).
- Intermittent apomorphine injections may be used to reduce 'off-time' in people with Parkinson's disease who have severe motor complications, though the evidence base is relatively poor. Side-effects including confusion and hallucinations can be a problem and there is a high incidence of injection-site reactions (Recommendation 48).
- Continuous subcutaneous infusions of apomorphine may be used to reduce 'off-time' and dyskinesia in people with Parkinson's disease who have severe motor complications, though the evidence base is relatively poor. Treatment should be initiated only in expert units with facilities for appropriate monitoring (Recommendation 49).
- It is not possible to identify a universal first-choice adjuvant drug therapy for treating later Parkinson's disease. The choice of adjuvant drug first prescribed should take into account:
  - clinical and lifestyle characteristics
  - patient preference, after the patient has been informed of the short-term and long-term benefits and drawbacks of the drug classes (Recommendation 50).

- To avoid the risk of acute akinesia or neuroleptic malignant syndrome, anti-parkinsonian medication should not be withdrawn abruptly or allowed to fail suddenly as a result of poor absorption (for example due to gastroenteritis, abdominal surgery) (Recommendation 51).
- The practice of so-called 'drug holidays', where anti-parkinsonian drugs are withdrawn in an attempt to reduce motor complications, should not be undertaken due to the risk of precipitating neuroleptic malignant syndrome (Recommendation 52).
- When patients with Parkinson's disease are admitted to hospital or care homes, it is important that their medication is:
  - given at the appropriate times (for some patients, self-medication may be appropriate)
  - only adjusted by, or after discussion with, a specialist in the management of Parkinson's disease.

  This reduces the risks associated with sudden changes in anti-parkinsonian medication (Recommendation 53).
- Clinicians should be aware of dopamine dysregulation syndrome. This is an uncommon disorder in which dopaminergic medication misuse is associated with abnormal behaviours, including hypersexuality, pathological gambling and stereotypic motor acts. When it occurs, this syndrome can be difficult to manage (Recommendation 54).

Surgery for Parkinson's disease

- Bilateral stimulation of the subthalamic nucleus (STN) may be used in people with Parkinson's disease who:
  - have motor complications that are refractory to best medical treatment
  - are biologically fit with no clinically significant active comorbidity
  - are levodopa responsive and
  - have no clinically significant active mental health problems, for example depression or dementia (Recommendation 55).
- Bilateral stimulation of the globus pallidus interna (GPi) may be used in people with Parkinson's disease who:
  - have motor complications that are refractory to best medical treatment
  - are biologically fit with no clinically significant active comorbidity
  - are levodopa responsive and
  - have no clinically significant active mental health problems, for example depression or dementia (Recommendation 56).

- At the present time there is insufficient evidence to determine whether stimulation of the STN or of the GPi is preferable. There is also insufficient evidence to determine whether one form of surgery is more effective or safer than the other. Observational studies suggest that stimulation of the STN may lead to better improvement in motor scores and more reduction in levodopa dose and depression scores, whereas stimulation of the GPi may lead to less cognitive impairment. When considering the type of surgery, it is recommended that account be taken of:
  - clinical and lifestyle characteristics of the person with Parkinson's disease
  - patient preference after the patient has been informed of the potential benefits and drawbacks of the different surgical procedures (Recommendation 57).
- In the UK, thalamic deep brain stimulation has been largely superseded by stimulation of the STN. Thalamic stimulation effectively reduces tremor, but the surgery is associated with risks of serious complications including cerebral infarction and haemorrhage. It is recommended that thalamic deep brain stimulation be considered as an option in people with Parkinson's disease in whom severe disabling tremor is the predominant symptom and where stimulation of the STN cannot be performed (Recommendation 58).

Non-motor features of Parkinson's disease

- Clinicians should have a low threshold for diagnosing depression in Parkinson's disease (Recommendation 59).
- There are difficulties in diagnosing mild depression in people with Parkinson's disease because the clinical features of depression can overlap with the motor features of the disease. Clinicians should be aware of this (Recommendation 60).
- The management of depression in people with Parkinson's disease should be tailored to the individual. It is important that account is taken of their co-existing therapy in order to avoid drug interactions (e.g. MAO-B inhibitors and antidepressants). Some antidepressants may make the motor symptoms of Parkinson's disease worse (Recommendation 61).
- All patients with Parkinson's disease and psychosis should receive a general medical evaluation and treatment for any precipitating condition (Recommendation 62).
- Consideration should be given to the gradual withdrawal of anti-parkinsonian medication that might have triggered psychosis in people with Parkinson's disease (Recommendation 63).

- If psychotic symptoms in people with Parkinson's disease are mild, they may not need to be actively treated, providing the patient (and carer) can tolerate them (Recommendation 64).
- Older (typical) antipsychotic drugs such as phenothiazines and butyrophenones should not be used in people with Parkinson's disease. They can exacerbate the motor features of the disease (Recommendation 65).
- Atypical antipsychotics may be considered for treatment of psychotic symptoms in people with Parkinson's disease. However, there is only limited evidence for their efficacy and safety in these patients (Recommendation 66).
- Clozapine may be used in the treatment of psychotic symptoms in Parkinson's disease, but registration with a monitoring scheme is required to detect the uncommon but potentially life-threatening complication of agranulocytosis. Few specialists caring for people with Parkinson's disease have experience with clozapine (Recommendation 67).
- Cholinesterase inhibitors have been used successfully in some patients for treating both cognitive decline and psychosis in Parkinson's disease dementia. Since a significant number of patients do not respond to this form of treatment, regular review is necessary to confirm its value. Further research is recommended to identify those patients who will benefit from this treatment (Recommendation 68).
- Sleep problems are common in Parkinson's disease and manifest in a variety of ways. A full sleep history should be taken from people with Parkinson's disease who report sleep disturbance (Recommendation 69).
- Good sleep hygiene should be advised in people with Parkinson's disease with any sleep disturbance. This includes:
  - the avoidance of stimulants (for example coffee, tea, caffeine) in the evening
  - establishing a regular pattern of sleep
  - ensuring bedding and temperature are comfortable
  - providing aids, such as a bed lever or rails to help with moving and turning, allowing the person to get more comfortable
  - restricting daytime siestas
  - giving advice about taking regular and appropriate exercise to induce better sleep
  - reviewing all medication and avoiding any drugs that may affect sleep or alertness, or may interact with other medication. Examples include selegiline, antihistamines, H_2-antagonists, antipsychotics and sedatives (Recommendation 70).
- It is important to identify and manage restless leg syndrome (RLS) and

rapid eye movement (REM) sleep behaviour disorder in people with Parkinson's disease and sleep disturbance (Recommendation 71).

- People with Parkinson's disease who have sudden onset of sleep should be advised not to drive and to consider any occupational hazards. Their medication should be adjusted if possible to reduce the occurrence of this effect (Recommendation 72).

- Although there is little evidence from trials of the efficacy and safety of modafinil in treating daytime hypersomnolence in Parkinson's disease, this drug may be considered for daytime hypersomnolence (Recommendation 73).

- Modified-release levodopa preparations may be used for nocturnal akinesia in people with Parkinson's disease (Recommendation 74).

- For all people with Parkinson's disease at risk of falling, a thorough assessment of the specific and non-specific predictors of falls together with the intrinsic and extrinsic factors that contribute to falls should be undertaken. The NICE clinical guideline number 21. *Falls: assessment and prevention of falls in older people* should be referred to (Recommendation 75).

- People with Parkinson's disease should be treated appropriately for the following autonomic disturbances:
  - urinary dysfunction (up to three-quarters of patients with Parkinson's disease develop bladder problems. Nocturia is the earliest and most common problem, although daytime urgency and frequency can also be troublesome. Urinary incontinence is common in Parkinson's disease)
  - weight loss (unintended weight loss is common in Parkinson's disease)
  - dysphagia (which increases the risks of asphyxiation, aspiration pneumonia, malnutrition and dehydration)
  - constipation (if caused by colonic dysmotility treatment should follow a staged, or stepladder, approach:
    - increasing dietary fibre and fluid intake, taking at least eight glasses of water per day and avoiding bananas
    - increasing exercise
    - fibre supplements such as psyllium or methylcellulose
    - stool softener (e.g. docusate sodium)
    - osmotic laxative (e.g. lactulose)
    - polyethylene glycol electrolyte-balanced solutions
    - occasional enemas (when required)
  - erectile dysfunction (is common in Parkinson's disease. Men with Parkinson's disease may also experience sexual dissatisfaction and

premature ejaculation. Women may experience difficulties with arousal, low sexual desire and anorgasmia)

- orthostatic hypotension (may contribute to falling; symptoms may include fatigue, pre-syncope and syncope)
- excessive sweating (severe sweating can occur as an end-of-dose off phenomenon or while in the 'on' motor state, usually associated with dyskinesias)
- sialorrhoea (excessive saliva or drooling occurs in up to 80% of people with Parkinson's disease; it seems to be more common in men) (Recommendation 76).

Other key interventions

- People with Parkinson's disease should have regular access to the following:
  - clinical monitoring and medication adjustment
  - a continuing point of contact for support, including home visits when appropriate
  - a reliable source of information about clinical and social matters of concern to people with Parkinson's disease and their carers, which may be provided by a Parkinson's disease nurse specialist (Recommendation 77).
- There is encouraging evidence from various trials of the effectiveness of some of the physiotherapy interventions suitable for people with Parkinson's disease. Physiotherapy services should be available for people with Parkinson's disease, with particular consideration given to:
  - gait re-education, improvement of balance and flexibility
  - enhancement of aerobic capacity
  - improvement of movement initiation
  - improvement of functional independence, including mobility and activities of daily living
  - provision of advice regarding safety in the home environment (Recommendation 78).
- The Alexander technique may be offered to benefit people with Parkinson's disease by helping them to make lifestyle adjustments that affect both the physical nature of the condition and the person's attitudes to having Parkinson's disease (Recommendation 79).
- Occupational therapy should be available for people with Parkinson's disease. Particular consideration should be given to:
  - maintaining work and family roles, home care and leisure activities
  - improving and maintaining patient transfers and mobility

- improving personal self-care activities such as eating, drinking, washing and dressing
- environmental issues to improve safety and motor function
- cognitive assessment and appropriate intervention (Recommendation 80).

- Speech and language therapy should be available for people with Parkinson's disease. Particular consideration should be given to:
  - improving vocal loudness and pitch range, including speech therapy programmes such as the Lee Silverman Voice Treatment (LSVT)
  - teaching strategies to optimise speech intelligibility
  - ensuring an effective means of communication is maintained throughout the course of the disease, including use of assistive technologies
  - review and management to support the safety and efficiency of swallowing and to minimise the risk of aspiration (Recommendation 81).

Palliative care in Parkinson's disease

- The needs of patients in the palliative care stage of Parkinson's disease are often under-recognised, and when they are it is often too late in the patient's care. Palliative care requirements of people with Parkinson's disease should be considered throughout all phases of the disease (Recommendation 82).
- People with Parkinson's disease and their carers should be given the opportunity to discuss end-of-life issues with appropriate healthcare professionals (Recommendation 83).

Community Pharmacy Parkinson's Disease Project

The European Parkinson's Disease Association (EPDA) proposed that a project should be carried out to find ways of reducing the problems patients have with medicines for their Parkinson's disease. The frequent adjustments in dosage, occurrence of adverse effects and a lack of understanding by patients about their medication often leads to suboptimal treatment and reduced compliance. The EPDA felt that community pharmacists with special expertise in Parkinson's disease and its management could provide a new type of service to these patients, with a view to improving the quality of their care and likely clinical outcome. Medicines Partnership, an initiative to improve concordance and compliance funded by the government, collaborated with the EPDA and other organisations and took the lead in setting the project up. Three primary care trusts (St Helen's, Brighton & Hove City, and Coventry PCTs) were selected in England to take part, and within each of these a number of community pharmacists were identified to provide the proposed new service. The next step was to provide specialist training to pharmacists taking part, in order to give them the necessary level of specialist knowledge and expertise. The specialist training consisted of 25 h covering clinical aspects, consultation skills, and service delivery.

Organisations involved

A number of organisations were involved with the project and all of those referred to below were represented on the steering group. Although the EPDA put forward the initial idea for the project, Medicines Partnership oversaw and co-ordinated it. Pharmacy Alliance worked with the Health Services Research Unit at the University of Oxford in designing and developing the service; this unit also evaluated the results. Pharmacy Alliance provided the training for the participating pharmacists and gave support to PCT co-ordinators. The specialist training material on the neurological aspects of the disease was provided by the Centre for Postgraduate Pharmacy Education. The Department of Health gave advice on the project and looked at the broader implications of the results, while the National Pharmaceutical Association focused on assessing the implications for community pharmacy. The Royal Pharmaceutical Society of Great Britain assessed the implications relating to the role of pharmacists. A substantial proportion of the funding for the project was provided by Pfizer. The membership of the steering group also included a number of specialists and a patient.

Recruitment

Patients were recruited into the project in a number of ways. Neurologists with patients in the geographical areas covered by the project wrote to them inviting participation. In addition, the project was publicised at local GP surgeries, neurology clinics and branch meetings of the Parkinson's Disease Society. Pharmacists taking part in the project were also able to recruit patients directly if they presented to the pharmacy. All patients were required to complete a baseline questionnaire and consent form, which were returned to the evaluation team.

Consultations

Over the next 6 months the pharmacists provided regular consultation for Parkinson's patients (and/or their carers) recruited into the study. During these consultations, patients had an opportunity to discuss their views and experiences with their medication, as well as any concerns they had about the condition. The pharmacists provided support and counselling on how the drug therapy worked, its side-effects and potential interactions. Help was also provided in optimising dosage timing and, if appropriate, practical aids were provided to reduce problems with drug administration. Dietary advice was also given. If problems were identified that the pharmacists were unable to address in the pharmacy, they would refer the patient back to their GP. If a pharmacist felt that the drug therapy should be changed, they would make recommendations to the GP or specialist. The consultation guide and form completed during the consultation with the patient or their carer is reproduced in Figure 8.1 (pages 162–164).

Evaluation

The project was evaluated at the Health Services Research Unit at the University of Oxford, and the results published in the summer of 2007.[35] Validated questionnaires were completed by patients or their carers, and focus groups were held consisting of selected participating patients and pharmacists. Three questionnaires were used: the Parkinson's Disease Questionnaire (PDQ 39) – a widely used disease-specific quality-of-life instrument; a questionnaire enabling assessment using a Satisfaction with Information on Medicines Scale (SIMS);[36] and one providing a measure on the Medicine Adherence Report Scale (MARS).[37]

The key aspects assessed included:

- patient satisfaction (with particular emphasis on the information they received about their medication and their understanding of their medicines)
- incidence of problems associated with medication (this included the occurrence of adverse effects or problems such as difficulty in swallowing medicines)
- health-related quality of life
- demands made upon other parts of the healthcare system
- degree of compliance with the agreed treatment regimen
- amount the service was used, and the experiences patients/carers had when using the service

Parkinson's Disease Consultation Guide

Patient ID Code: _____ Pharmacy ID Code: _____ Date: _____

| Recruitment | **OR** | Follow-up | Did the patient present with an ID Code?: Yes | **OR** | No | Domiciliary visit?: Yes | **OR** | No |

This consultation guide should be **completed by the pharmacist**, during the consultation with the patient/carer.

- Thank the patient for agreeing to participate in the Parkinson's Disease programme.
- Explain the purpose of the programme and that you will ask them a series of questions in relation to their condition and its treatment.
- **For example**: " *I would like to ensure that you are getting maximum benefit from your medicines, and try to resolve any issues or concerns that you may have. Any responses you give me will be completely confidential.*"

Opening Questions – To be completed at FIRST VISIT ONLY

1. Patient Name: _____

2. Age: _____ **3. Sex:** Male **or** Female

4. Are you: Patient **or** Patient's carer

5. How long have you been diagnosed with Parkinson's Disease?

_____ months _____ years

6. Which of the following, if any, have you seen in the past 6 months regarding the management of your PD?

GP	Consultant neurologist
PD Nurse	Consultant geriatrician
Pharmacist	Consultant physician
Other	_____

(please state)

> **NOTE:** Start by obtaining full details of the patients' medication by completing a medication history form.

7. *"So, how have you been getting on with your PD medicines in general?"*

_____

_____

_____

	Yes	No	Some-times
a. Are you able to incorporate your medicine(s) into your normal day okay?			
b. Do you manage to take your PD medicines exactly as instructed?			
If NOT, why? _____			
c. How do you remember to take your PD medicines?			
d. Do you think your PD medications are working?			
e. Do you have problems with swallowing your PD medicines?			
f. Do you have problems with opening bottles/containers to access your PD medicines?			

Developed by Pharmacy Alliance and Medicines Partnership for the Community Pharmacy PD Programme – June 2004

8. Would you mind if I ask you a few questions now about how you are getting on with your Parkinson's Disease?

a. What is a typical day like for you, with PD?

b. What is the biggest challenge you face with your PD treatment?

c. Are you aware of any uncontrolled/unmanaged side-effects from your PD medicine(s)?

How often, during the past month have you...............	Never	Rarely	Some-times	Often	Always
9 Felt slow & stiff before your next dose of your PD medicine was due?					
10 Experienced episodes of 'freezing' (feel stuck to the spot and unable to move)?					
11 Noticed a change in your pattern/control, when passing urine?					
12 Experienced difficulty or pain on emptying your bowels?					
13 Experienced wriggling or writhing movements that you were unable to control, and that have been distressing to you?					
14 Noticed a significant decrease in body weight?					
15 Felt dizzy, light-headed or had a fall?					
16 Experienced difficulties with sleep-related problems? (e.g. nightmares, waking up in the night)					
17 Felt excessively sleepy or experienced sudden onset of sleep during the day?					
18 Felt low in spirit or depressed?					
19 Felt unusually anxious or agitated?					
20 Been more forgetful than usual or had difficulty remembering things?					
21 Had distressing hallucinations? (i.e. something you see, hear or feel that was not there)					
22 Felt nauseous or been sick?					
23 Experienced change in severity of pain in your muscles, joints or body?					

Developed by Pharmacy Alliance and Medicines Partnership for the Community Pharmacy PD Programme – June 2004

Information Needs

'I may be able to help you with any extra information you might need about your PD and it's treatment....'

24. Do you know what your PD medicines are for?

   Yes   No   Unsure

25. Do you know **HOW** and **WHEN** to take your PD medicines?

   Yes   No   Unsure

26. Do you know what to do if you miss a dose of your PD medication?

   Yes   No   Unsure

29. Do you have any other questions or concerns, regarding your PD and/or its treatment, that I may be able to help you with?

Questions/Notes

Date of next appointment:

Domiciliar visit   OR   **In Pharmacy**

How many **prescribed medicines** is the patient CURRENTLY taking to treat their **PD**?

How many **OTHER prescribed medicines** is the patient CURRENTLY taking?

Thank you for taking the time to participate in this programme. I will try to address your concerns or issues and answer any questions you may have. I will also arrange a follow-up date for you to return to the pharmacy to enable me to monitor your condition and your current treatments and to address any further questions or concerns you have.

Developed by Pharmacy Alliance and Medicines Partnership for the Community Pharmacy PD Programme – June 2004

Figure 8.1   Parkinson's disease consultation guide. Developed by the Pharmacy Alliance and Medicines Partnership for the Community Pharmacy PD Programme, June 2004.

- interventions and referrals made by pharmacists
- feedback on service (from patients/carers, pharmacists, GPs and other healthcare professionals involved)
- impact on participating pharmacists (in terms of their skills, knowledge and confidence).

Results

The authors of the formal evaluation carried out at the Health Services Research Unit at the University of Oxford,[35] concluded that the results are encouraging. During the 6-month study, a statistically significant improvement in self-reported health status on the physical functioning domain of the PDQ 39 was demonstrated. There was also a statistically significant improvement in the proportion of people indicating satisfaction with the information on what their medication does and on potential problems with medication as scored using the SIMS. However, no significant change occurred on the MARS.

A total of 336 patient consultations were conducted during the study, over 50% of these taking place within the community pharmacy and 40% in patients' homes. At the time of recruitment, more than 30% of patients believed that their medication was not working or felt that it was only working some of the time. More than one-third of patients admitted they sometimes forgot to take medication prescribed for their Parkinson's disease and one-third said they were either unsure or did not know what their medicines were for. One-quarter of patients at the start of the study stated they were not sure what they should do if they happened to miss a dose. Clearly these figures show there is a definite need for increasing the information, advice and support given to patients.

During consultations with the pharmacist the average calculated incidence of problems identified was 1.5 per consultation. The most frequent problems were:

- uncontrolled and unmanaged symptoms
- the occurrence of side-effects
- the need for review of dosage or treatment regimen.

Pharmacists taking part in the project made a total of 596 interventions, three-quarters of which were addressed by the pharmacist themselves and one-quarter were referred.

The feedback from patients at the end of the study was very positive.[38] More than 87% of patients considered the pharmacist to be knowledgeable about Parkinson's disease and would recommend the new service to others suffering with the condition. The advice given by the pharmacists was felt to be helpful by 82%, and 70% judged that they had gained greater benefits from their drug therapy since taking part in the study. More than 60% of patients considered they knew more about the disease and their treatment from the consultations. One view expressed by a patient was:

> I feel like I'm in the hands of the experts . . . like the pharmacist and neurologist.[38]

Clearly, the results of this project are encouraging and should be considered by commissioners of services when deciding how these should be delivered. With proposals for establishing pharmacists with special interests (PhwSIs) being announced by the Department of Health at around the same time as the above results, it is timely to explore this new initiative as a way of improving services and the care available to patients suffering with Parkinson's disease (see Plate 12).

Clinical pharmacy and pharmaceutical care issues

Drug therapy is a major component of the overall care of patients suffering with Parkinson's disease. The fact that medication regimens can be complex, often requiring fine tuning, and the high potential for the occurrence of adverse effects and interactions with other agents, makes this an area where good management of medicines use can have a major influence on the clinical outcome and wellbeing of patients. Much of the content of this book is highly relevant to the practice of clinical pharmacy and the provision of pharmaceutical care to patients. Chapter 3 gives detailed information on the approach to treatment and the use of anti-Parkinson's drugs, and appendices (B and C) are provided at the back of the book, which cover drug interactions and adverse effects. The treatment of a wide range of symptoms other than the effects of the disease on motor function is discussed in Chapter 6. The case study (page 170) provides an opportunity to practise addressing clinical pharmacy and pharmaceutical care issues with a clinical scenario. This will be particularly valuable for undergraduate students of pharmacy and pharmacists studying for postgraduate examinations.

Compliance and concordance

Much has been written about patients taking medicines and the factors that determine whether this is done in accordance with the intensions of the prescriber. Terms such as 'adherence' 'compliance', and in more recent years 'concordance' have been used, often incorrectly, to describe this aspect of medicine taking. Of course, the assumption that patient compliance with medication instructions will always result in optimal care is an incorrect one. It ignores the possibility of deficiencies elsewhere in the various stages of decision making which, although aimed at maximising the chance of best clinical outcome, may not always do so.[39] Pharmaceutical care must focus on all steps leading to, and involving the use of drug therapy, including the assessment of outcomes, both beneficial and harmful.

Involving patients in decision making and helping them to better understand the use of medicines and what to expect from their effects, is not only something which patients increasingly want, but is also helpful to all concerned. Good communication is essential to facilitate this, and special efforts may be needed when discussing treatment with patients who have Parkinson's disease, since the condition may sometimes compromise communication. A patient's speech may be affected, and altered body language (e.g. bland facial expression) may hamper dialogue, and healthcare professionals must take this into account. Pharmacists involved with the pharmaceutical care of these patients must maximise their listening skills and their effectiveness at imparting information and advice in order to successfully create two-way communication between themselves and patient. By ensuring that patients *understand* their medication (and are not just given information about it), the chance of maximising its potential benefits is increased. A patient who feels there is good rapport between themself and the pharmacist is more likely to allude to any problems or worries they have, and indicate changes that have occurred that may signal the need for a review of medication.

In addition to the need for patient understanding and concordance, pharmacists should consider the practicalities of drug therapy for patients with Parkinson's disease. Amongst other things, this includes considering compliance aids, which may be helpful for some patients, especially those with later-stage disease. Potential physical obstacles to successful medicine taking include difficulties a patient can have in pressing tablets or capsules from foil strips, or problems opening containers.

Drug therapy during hospital admissions

Hospital pharmacists have long recognised the problem of loss in symptom control, which can occur when patients with Parkinson's disease are admitted to hospital. Often this is due to them no longer receiving their medication at the times they have been used to. In many cases, patients have ascertained what works best for themselves, but then find that the ward routine disrupts this, for example drug rounds may be timed differently from the patient's normal pattern of drug administration.

In 2006, the Parkinson's Disease Society ran a campaign highlighting the problems that can arise following hospital admission. The society recognised that many patients and their families were worried about the prospect of hospital stays or respite care. Much of their anxiety is caused by their belief (often well founded) that professionals involved in their care will not understand the challenges they face living with Parkinson's disease and the need for maintaining certain routines such as drug-administration schedules. Staff on wards that do not specialise in neurology or care of the elderly often do not appreciate that therapy has been tailored to the individual patient in order to gain maximum benefit and best quality of life. It is often the case that deterioration in a patient's condition, for example increased 'off' time or more severe dyskinesia, is precipitated by changes in dosage forms or timing of medication, and it may not be recognised that this is the cause. The distress to the patient and relatives can be immense as activities of daily living such as eating, drinking, and mobility deteriorate. If a patient is able to self-medicate while in hospital this helps overcome the difficulty of inflexible drug rounds.

Hospital pharmacists should appreciate the risks of other drugs that may be administered during the patient's stay, either exacerbating symptoms of their condition or increasing the chance of adverse effects from therapy they are already taking. A large range of potential drug interactions can occur with medication for Parkinson's disease, and a careful assessment of the appropriateness of additional drug therapy should be made. It must be remembered that a serious interaction between selegiline and pethidine can occur, and therefore this commonly used analgesic should be avoided. Other commonly used drugs that may be contraindicated include metoclopramide, prochlorperazine, and other drugs that have the potential to cause drug-induced parkinsonism. Domperidone *is* suitable as an anti-emetic in patients with Parkinson's disease.

Pharmacists with special interest

The British Pharmaceutical Conference in Manchester (September 2006), saw the launch of the Department of Health's framework for establishing pharmacists with special interests (PhwSIs) (see Plate 12).[40] The minister of state for delivery and quality explained to the audience how the framework should build on pharmacists' core roles, and provides commissioners with an opportunity to maximise the contribution pharmacists can make in specialist areas to ensure patients received the highest quality of care. The minister indicated that the concept is applicable not only to the community and other primary care-based pharmacists, but to hospital pharmacists as well. Within the hospital sector, pharmacists also have the opportunity to specialise by becoming consultant pharmacists. Since drug therapy plays a major part in the management of Parkinson's disease, this therapeutic area would seem particularly suitable for pharmacists specialising in the condition. The results of the Community Pharmacist Parkinson's Disease Project (see page 165) reinforce this view.

Community pharmacy contractual framework

In April 2005 the Department of Health announced a new contractual framework for NHS community pharmacy services.[41] This has increased the range of services that pharmacists can offer, including support to people suffering with long-term conditions. Three categories of services are included in the framework:

- essential services
- advanced services
- enhanced services.

The advanced services include medicines use review (MUR). Enhanced services are those that PCTs commission locally to meet the needs of the local population. Both of these create the opportunity for providing better support for patients with respect to their drug therapy. Since long-term conditions are specifically cited in the Department of Health document, it would seem the framework would be particularly suitable for patients with Parkinson's disease.

The Department of Health has given examples of enhanced services that PCTs can commission pharmacists to provide. These include setting up clinics for people with long-term conditions. Although diabetes is used to illustrate this, the idea is just as applicable to Parkinson's disease. The provision of MUR (under the category of advanced services) is stated in the document 'to improve support for people who have long-term conditions by spotting and resolving problems with medication at an early stage, so helping to reduce hospital admissions'.[41]

Community pharmacy services may also develop roles as a result of practice-based commissioning whereby GPs enter into agreements with local pharmacists around service provision. The general medical services contract for GPs includes standards for medicines management. The specification for medication reviews, which need to be done every 15 months to meet the standard, states that these may be carried out by a pharmacist. Pharmacists are well placed to undertake this role since it combines their clinical knowledge and skills of therapeutics and counselling with product knowledge and medication supply. There is good evidence that medication reviews carried out by pharmacists who have access to the necessary patient records, benefit patients and the NHS.[42] Full access to medical records is vital if reviews are to be successful. At present this is usually only practical if pharmacists carry out reviews in doctors' surgeries. There are examples where this is now happening. A GP practice of 12 GPs in Hampstead, north London, has commissioned a community pharmacist to hold sessions at the surgery undertaking reviews for patients aged over 65 years who are taking four or more medicines.[43] Until better access to electronic patient records becomes available, this seems the obvious way to proceed.

CASE STUDY

Readers are invited to read the brief outline below and then give consideration to the issues raised in the table that follows. Those studying for examinations in medicine or pharmacy may find this particularly useful and are urged to attempt the questions raised in the right-hand column of the table before proceeding to the following pages which suggest appropriate answers and explanations.

Mr Williams

Mr Williams is 57 years old and has been a taxi driver for 32 years. For some months now, he has noticed that his right hand trembles, especially in the evening when he is relaxing watching the television. This effect seems to disappear when using the hand, but the trembling often re-appears when his hand is resting on his lap. Mr Williams mentioned this to his GP when visiting him for a routine review of his medication for hypertension, which is fairly well controlled.

The GP observes the tremor, noticing that it is only apparent in the right hand and that it stops when the hand is performing some action such as picking up a pen from the desk. Although not mentioning the possible diagnosis, he is wondering whether Mr Williams is showing the early stages of Parkinson's disease and refers him to the neurology clinic at the local hospital.

Mr Williams is given an appointment to see a neurologist 5 weeks later. After taking a medical history and examining the patient, the neurologist informs him that he thinks it very likely he has the early stages of Parkinson's disease. He arranges a blood test and fixes another appointment to see Mr Williams in 3 weeks' time to discuss the diagnosis further.

1.	Although the GP suspects Parkinson's disease, he does not indicate this and refers Mr Williams to the neurology clinic.	Why would the GP refrain from making a firm diagnosis of Parkinson's disease there and then?
	At the first appointment with the neurologist, a blood test is arranged for Mr Williams.	What is the value of the blood test?
2.	The patient is a 57-year-old taxi driver. His symptoms are mild and not considered by the patient to be particularly troublesome.	What issues need to be considered?
		Suggest a course of action for this stage of Parkinson's disease.
3.	The patient is now 58 years old, the symptoms are troubling him and pramipexole is started.	Does this seem a reasonable choice of drug?
		What would be an appropriate regimen for establishing therapy with pramipexole?
		Outline any side-effect issues that may be of concern.
4.	The patient is now 60 years old and retired. Co-careldopa is added as symptoms have become much more severe. The patient is complaining of nausea and occasional vomiting (assumed to be due to the new drug).	What measures can be tried to improve tolerance to the drug?
		If an anti-emetic is to be used, which one would be most suitable?
5.	The patient is now 67 years old. The dose of co-careldopa has increased over the years. The patient is experiencing persistent 'end-of-dose' wearing-off effects and selegiline is added.	What is the rationale for adding selegiline?
		How does selegiline work?

continued overleaf

Case Study (continued)

6.	The patient is now 68 years old. He goes to his GP complaining of depression, who prescribes fluoxetine.	Comment on the occurrence of depression in this patient.
		Would you anticipate any problems with the use of fluoxetine; if yes, what is the nature of the risk?
7.	The patient is now 69 years old and has developed motor complications (dyskinesia) from the levodopa.	What drug might be helpful in reducing this problem?
8.	The patient is now 73 years old and is achieving only poor control with his current drug therapy. Symptoms are now severely disabling.	Which injectable drug for treating Parkinson's disease might be worth trying?
		In what ways can this be administered?
		What are the potential problems with this form of therapy and how can these be minimised?

1. **Although the GP suspects Parkinson's disease, he refrains from making a diagnosis, but refers the patients to a neurologist. During the first appointment at the neurology clinic a blood test is arranged.**

Diagnosis of Parkinson's disease

The diagnosis of Parkinson's disease can sometimes be difficult. Even experienced neurologists and physicians specialising in the care of the elderly make an incorrect diagnosis in a proportion of patients; it has been suggested misdiagnosis occurs in around 10% of cases. The incidence of misdiagnosis by GPs is obviously higher. A number of syndromes have a similar presentation to that of true Parkinson's disease. Parkinsonian symptoms can also be caused by a number of drugs, other conditions such as essential tremor or hyperthyroidism. An accurate diagnosis is important as it affects prognosis and treatment. The Guidelines published in 2006 state that a patient with suspected Parkinson's disease should be referred *quickly* and *untreated* to a specialist with expertise in the differential diagnosis of this condition.[32] If the symptoms are mild, the patient should be seen within 6 weeks, but new referrals in later disease with more complex problems should be seen within 2 weeks. The GP should not initiate any therapy since this may complicate the process of diagnosis by a specialist.

The value of blood tests

The diagnosis of Parkinson's disease is primarily based on clinical signs and symptoms, but blood tests can be helpful in ruling out other conditions producing similar symptoms. For example, hyperthyroidism can produce tremor; this condition can be easily ruled out. Had the patient been younger (less than 50 years of age), a blood test to eliminate Wilson's disease is considered essential by many neurologists. Serum caeruloplasmin and measurement of levels of copper in urine enable this.

2. **The patient is a 57-year-old taxi driver whose symptoms are mild and not considered by the patient to be particularly troublesome.**

Issues to be considered

The patient should be provided with details about the disease, including prognosis and treatments, and reassurance given as necessary. This must be done skilfully with honesty, while maintaining a positive outlook. Details of further sources of information and support should be given.

In the early days of Parkinson's disease, drug therapy is often unnecessary. However, most patients will deteriorate to a point where, within 2 years of diagnosis, drug therapy is needed. Some patients with mild symptoms such as just a tremor in one arm may carry on for much longer without the need to start drug therapy.

All drugs used to treat Parkinson's disease have the potential to cause adverse effects. These can be more troublesome than the symptoms the patient has and are occasionally serious, so treatment is not normally commenced until the patient begins to experience functional difficulties.

There is no evidence that starting drug therapy early will slow down or delay disease progression. Treatment is symptomatic and is aimed at improving the ability of patients to maintain activities of daily living, and function and work as normally as possible. These in turn help retain good quality of life.

A particular anxiety this patient is likely to have is whether he can continue driving. Certainly there are important issues especially once drug therapy is started. Many of the drugs have been associated with daytime sleepiness and sudden onset of sleep, particularly levodopa and dopamine receptor agonists. The Parkinson's disease itself may reduce driving skills and obviously there exists a major responsibility for ensuring the safety of the patient, any passengers and other road users. The patient should inform the

continued overleaf

DVLA of the condition at the time of diagnosis, and their insurance company (see Appendix D).

Course of action at this stage

Ensure an explanation on all the issues above is given. Drug therapy is not appropriate yet. Monitor and review the patient's condition at appropriate intervals.

3.   **Now 58 years old, the symptoms are troubling him and pramipexole is started.**

Choice of drug

Many neurologists would consider a non-ergot dopamine agonist to be the most appropriate drug in this case. Dopamine agonists cause fewer problems with dyskinesias and are often effective as monotherapy in the early stages of Parkinson's disease when symptoms are still mild but sufficiently troublesome to warrant treatment. This approach is also considered particularly suitable for younger patients with the disease.

Pramipexole treatment regimen

- Week 1: 88 μg three times daily
- Week 2: 180 μg three times daily
- Week 3: 350 μg three times daily
  (These dosages are expressed in terms of milligrams of salt)
- Thereafter:
  - the daily dose can be increased by 540 μg at weekly intervals if necessary to achieve maximal therapeutic effect, providing the patient does not experience unacceptable side-effects
  - the maximum daily dose is 3.3 mg in divided doses.
    If it becomes necessary to stop treatment with pramipexole, this should be done gradually.

Side-effects

A wide range of side-effects can occur (as with all drugs used in the treatment of Parkinson's disease). Nausea is very common and occurs in approximately 1 in 6 patients. Other common side-effects include dyskinesia, constipation, fatigue, headache, somnolence, confusion, hallucinations (particularly visual) and insomnia. Sudden onset of sleep is uncommon, but presents a particular risk especially if a patient is driving or undertaking other activities that require constant alertness. Hypotension can occur, especially in the early days of treatment. This side-effect is more likely if the dosage is increased too rapidly. Because of the risk, albeit low, of visual disorders, regular ophthalmological testing is recommended.

4.   **Now 60 years old and retired, the patient's symptoms are much worse and co-careldopa is added. The patient is complaining of nausea and occasional vomiting (assumed to be due to the new drug).**

Improving tolerance to the drug

Nausea and vomiting are associated with the use of co-careldopa and co-beneldopa. However, occasionally, changing from one to the other improves severe gastrointestinal symptoms.

Taking the dose with a little food (e.g. light snack) is found by some patients to reduce side-effects.

Altering the regimen so smaller doses are taken after food may be a suitable approach for some patients.

Choice of anti-emetic

Domperidone can be taken to reduce nausea and vomiting. This anti-emetic does not block the effects of dopamine inside the brain so is not contraindicated in patients with Parkinson's disease.

5.   **The patient is now 67 years old. The dose of co-careldopa has increased over the years. The patient is experiencing persistent 'end-of-dose' wearing-off effects and selegiline is added.**

Rationale for adding selegiline

Selegiline has been found to be effective in reducing the 'end-of-dose' wearing-off effect that often occurs with more advanced Parkinson's disease. Some believe the buccal formulation of selegiline to be more effective than the standard formulation in helping with motor fluctuations in people with later Parkinson's disease.

Mode of action of selegiline

Selegiline is a monoamine oxidase-B inhibitor which reduces the breakdown of dopamine in neurons. As a result, higher concentrations of the transmitter are available at synaptic level.

continued overleaf

Case Study (continued)

6. **The patient is now 68 years old. He visits the GP complaining that he feels quite depressed. The GP has prescribed fluoxetine to treat this.**

Depression in Parkinson's disease

Depression is commonly associated with Parkinson's disease. Often patients complain that they do not sleep so well and wake up earlier than they used to in the mornings. Increased feelings of sadness and being helpless frequently occur, and what may appear to be signs of worsening Parkinson's disease such as increased tremor and further slowing in movement, may in fact be due to depression. It has been estimated that the mean prevalence of depression in patients with Parkinson's disease is around 40%. It is important that the effect on quality of life from this symptom is not underestimated. For many patients this may be a more significant problem than the motor impairment that they experience.

The use of fluoxetine in this patient

Fluoxetine is a selective serotonin reuptake inhibitor (SSRI) antidepressant. This patient is currently taking selegiline for the persistent 'end-of-dose' wearing-off effects that he was experiencing with his levodopa therapy. There are a number of reports of a potentially serious interaction occurring when fluoxetine is taken by patients receiving selegiline. In fact, it is recommended that a patient in whom fluoxetine is to be commenced, stops their selegiline for 2 weeks beforehand. In the reverse situation, i.e. if a patient is already taking fluoxetine, this should be stopped for 5 weeks before commencing treatment with selegiline. The interaction can result in CNS excitation and hypertension. (Note: this patient is already receiving drug therapy for high blood pressure.) In one published report, a patient's blood pressure rose to 200/120 mmHg, her hands became blue and the patient experienced episodes of shivering and sweating after a few days of starting fluoxetine 20 mg.[44] She was taking selegiline for her Parkinson's disease. When the selegiline and fluoxetine were stopped the adverse effects resolved. Fluoxetine was later restarted (without restarting the selegiline) with no untoward effects. Other effects have been reported when the two drugs are used together, including hyperactivity, manic behaviour, confusion, ataxia, headache, flushes, palpitations and tonic–clonic seizures. The mechanism for the interaction is unclear, but in many ways it is consistent with the so-called serotonin syndrome. The interaction does not manifest in everyone; some patients have taken the combination with no adverse effect. However, given the nature and severity of the potential effects, the concomitant use of these drugs is not recommended.

7.   The patient is now 69 years old and has developed motor complications (dyskinesia) from the levodopa.

Drug therapy for treating dyskinesias

Amantadine is not itself a particularly effective agent for the treatment of Parkinson's disease; however, it is useful in treating dyskinesias that are particularly troublesome in later stages of the disease. There is a lack of data on its long-term benefits; there is some evidence that its anti-dyskinetic effect reduces substantially after a few months of therapy.

8.   The patient is now 73 years old and is achieving only poor control with his current drug therapy. Symptoms are now severely disabling.

Injectable drug therapy for treating severely disabling Parkinson's disease

Apomorphine injection is only used in advanced disease in patients who have major problems with 'off' periods despite optimising treatment with levodopa.

Methods of administration

Currently, apomorphine can only be administered by injection, though the intranasal and other routes are the subject of research. It cannot be given orally since substantial first-pass metabolism in the liver results in very low bioavailability. The drug is injected subcutaneously, but frequent injections may be necessary throughout the day. If more than ten injections daily are needed, administration by subcutaneous infusion via a pump is likely to be preferable.

Problems with apomorphine therapy

Treatment with apomorphine requires expertise and should only be initiated by specialist centres. Hospital admission is necessary when starting a patient on this form of therapy, and it is crucial that ongoing provision of support is available when the patient returns home. Clearly, injecting the drug or setting up a portable infusion pump can cause practical difficulties, and family or carers may need to assist with this.

The drug is highly emetogenic and at least 2 days' treatment with domperidone is necessary before commencing apomorphine, to reduce the problem of nausea and vomiting.

As with other dopamine agonists, adverse effects are common and include confusion, drowsiness, postural hypotension and hallucinations. Injection site

continued overleaf

Case Study (continued)

reactions are often a problem and can lead to the formation of nodules and ulceration. It is important that different injection sites are used by the patient to reduce this risk.

References

1. Department of Health. *The National Service Framework for Long Term Conditions*. London: Department of Health, 2005. www.dh.gov.uk/en/ Publicationsandstatistics/Publications/PublicationsPolicyAndGuidance/DH_4 105361 (accessed 7 June 2007).
2. Department of Health. *The NHS Improvement Plan: putting people at the heart of public services*. Cm 6268. London: HMSO, 2004. www.dh.gov.uk/ prod_consum_dh/groups/dh_digitalassets/@dh/@en/documents/digitalasset/ dh_4084522.pdf (accessed 7 June 2007).
3. Department of Health. *National Standards, Local Action: Health and Social Care Standards and Planning Framework 2005/6–2007/8*. London: The Stationery Office, 2003.
4. www.modern.nhs.uk/action-on (accessed 7 June 2007).
5. The Modernisation Agency/Department of Health. *Neuroscience Critical Care Report – Progress in Developing Services*. London: Department of Health, 2004. www.wise.nhs.uk/sites/clinicalimprovcollab/cc/Background %20Information/1/Neuroscience%20Critical%20Care%20Report%20 %20Progress%20in%20Developing%20Services%20(August%202004).pdf (accessed 7 June 2007).
6. Department of Health. *Long Term Conditions CGWT*. www.dh.gov.uk/ PolicyAndGuidance/HumanResourcesAndTraining/ModernisingWorkforce-PlanningHome/CGWTLongTerm/fs/en (accessed 7 June 2007).
7. Department of Health. *Making a Difference. Strengthening the nursing, midwifery and health visiting contribution to health and healthcare*. London: Department of Health, 1999. www.dh.gov.uk/en/Publicationsandstatistics/ Lettersandcirculars/Healthservicecirculars/DH_4004153 (accessed 7 June 2007).
8. Department of Health. *Developing Key Roles for Nurses and Midwives – a Guide for Managers*. London: Department of Health, 2002. www.dh.gov.uk/ en/Publicationsandstatistics/Publications/PublicationsPolicyAndGuidance/ DH_4009527 (accessed 16 July 2007).
9. Department of Health. *The NHS Plan: a plan for investment a plan for reform*. Cm 4818-I. Norwich: HMSO, 2000. www.dh.gov.uk/en/Publications andstatistics/Publications/PublicationsPolicyAndGuidance/DH_4002960 (accessed 7 June 2007).
10. Department of Health. *Liberating the Talents: helping primary care trusts and nurses to deliver the NHS Plan*. London: Department of Health, 2002. www. dh.gov.uk/en/Publicationsandstatistics/Publications/PublicationsPolicyAnd Guidance/DH_4007473 (accessed 7 June 2007).

11. www.dh.gov.uk/nurseprescribing (accessed 7 June 2007).
12. www.dh.gov.uk/supplementaryprescribing (accessed 7 June 2007).
13. www.groupprotocols.org.uk (accessed 7 June 2007).
14. Department of Health. *Meeting the Challenge: a strategy for the allied health professions.* London: Department of Health, 2000. www.dh.gov.uk/en/Publicationsandstatistics/Publications/PublicationsPolicyAndGuidance/DH_4 025477 (accessed 7 June 2007).
15. Department of Health. *The Chief Health Professions Officer's Ten Key Roles for Allied Health Professionals.* London: Department of Health, 2003. www.dh.gov.uk/prod_consum_dh/groups/dh_digitalassets/@dh/@en/documents/digitalasset/dh_4061612.pdf (accessed 16 July 2007).
16. www.dh.gov.uk/en/Policyandguidance/Medicinespharmacyandindustry/Prescriptions/TheNon-MedicalPrescribingProgramme/Supplementary prescribing/index.htm (accessed 16 July 2007).
17. NATPACT AHP Significant Issues Group. *Allied Health Professionals Self-Assessment Tool.) Self-Assessment Tool for AHPs.* London: NHS Modernisation Agency, 2003. www.natpact.nhs.uk/uploads/aph_framework.pdf (accessed 7 June 2007).
18. Department of Health. *A Vision for Pharmacy in the New NHS.* London: Department Of Health, 2003. www.dh.gov.uk/en/Consultations/Closedconsultations/DH_4068353 (accessed 16 July 2007).
19. Department of Health. *Community Prescribing by Pharmacists starts in England.* Press release 7 May 2004. www.dh.gov.uk/en/Publicationsand statistics/Pressreleases/DH_4081900 (accessed 16 July 2007). dh.gov.uk/PolicyAndGuidance/MedicinesPharmacyAndIndustryServices/Prescriptions/SupplementaryPrescribing/fs/en
20. Department of Health. *Implementing the New Community Pharmacy Contractual Framework (draft) – Information for Primary Care Trusts.* www.dh.gov.uk/en/Publicationsandstatistics/Publications/PublicationsPolicyAndGuidance/DH_4109256 (accessed 16 July 2007).
21. www.npc.co.uk/mms/index.htm (accessed 28 September 2007).
22. Department of Health. *Management of Medicines – a Resource to Support Implementation of the Wider Aspects of Medicines Management for the National Service Frameworks for Diabetes, Renal Services and Long-term Conditions.* London: Department of Health, 2004. www.dh.gov.uk/asset Root/04/08/87/55/04088755.pdf (accessed 7 June 2007).
23. Medicines Partnership and Department of Health. *Focus on your Medicines.* London: Medicines Partnership and Department of Health, 2004. www.npc.co.uk/med_partnership/medication-review/focus-on-your-medicines.html (accessed 7 June 2007).
24. Medicines Partnership and Department of Health. *Focus on your Health for people with Epilepsy.* London: Medicines Partnership and Department of Health, 2004.
25. www.msdecisions.org.uk (accessed 7 June 2007).
26. News feature: Parkinson's project ready for take-off. *Pharm J* 2004; 272: 442.
27. www.medguides.medicines.org.uk/ (accessed 7 June 2007).
28. Department of Health. *Policy Background – Practitioners with Special Interests (PwSIs).* www.dh.gov.uk/en/Policyandguidance/Organisationpolicy/

Primarycare/Practitionerswithspecialinterests/DH_4066010 (accessed 16 July 2007).

29. www.natpact.nhs.uk/cms/165.php (accessed 7 June 2007).

30. Department of Health. *Long-Term Conditions Information Strategy: supporting the National Service Framework for Long Term Conditions.* London: Department of Health, 2005. www.dh.gov.uk/en/Publicationsandstatistics/Publications/PublicationsPolicyAndGuidance/DH_4106014 (accessed 16 June 2007).

31. National Institute for Health and Clinical Excellence. *Clinical guideline 35. Parkinson's Disease: diagnosis and management in primary and secondary care.* London: NICE, 2006. www.nice.org.uk/CG035 (accessed 8 June 2007).

32. National Collaborating Centre for Chronic Conditions. *Parkinson's Disease: diagnosis and management in primary and secondary care* [full guideline]. London: National Collaborating Centre for Chronic Conditions, 2006. Available from the Royal College of Physicians website, www.rcplondon.ac.uk/pubs/brochure.aspx?e=34; the NICE website, www.nice.org.uk/CG035fullguideline; and the National Library for Health website, www.nlh.nhs.uk (accessed 8 June 2007).

33. National Institute for Health and Clinical Excellence. Quick reference guide N1052. *Parkinson's Disease: diagnosis and management in primary and secondary care.* London: NICE, 2006. www.nice.org.uk/CG035quickrefguide (accessed 8 June 2007).

34. National Institute for Health and Clinical Excellence. *Understanding NICE Guidance – information for people who use NHS services. Clinical guideline 35 Parkinson's disease.* www.nice.org.uk/CG035publicinfo (accessed 8 June 2007).

35. Mynors G, Jenkinson C, MacNeill V, Balcon R. A pilot evaluation of specialist community pharmacy services for patients with Parkinson's disease. *Pharm J* 2007; 278: 709–712.

36. Horne R, Hankins M, Jenkins R. The satisfaction with information about medicines scale (SIMS): a new measurement tool for audit and research. *Qual Health Care* 2001; 10: 135–140.

37. Horn R, Hankins M. *The Medicines Adherence Report Scale (MARS).* Brighton: University of Brighton, 2003.

38. Baker MG. *The Parkinson's Disease Pharmacy Project. Making better use of community pharmacy services.* Presentation at The European Parkinson's Disease Association Conference, London, May 2006. Patients and their medicines: optimising the outcomes. www.npc.co.uk/pdf/Mary_Baker.pdf (accessed 8 June 2007).

39. Webb D, Sanghani P, Tugwell C, Cross M. Concordance: last link in the chain? *Pharm J* 1999; 263: 782.

40. Department of Health. *Implementing Care Closer to Home – Providing Convenient Quality Care for Patients. A National Framework for Pharmacists with Special Interests.* London: Department of Health, 2006.

41. *Dawn of New Era for Pharmacy.* Press release, 2005/0151, Department of Health, 1 April 2005. www.dh.gov.uk/en/Publicationsandstatistics/Press releases/DH_4107503 (accessed 8 June 2007).

42. Petty D, Rayner DKT, Zermansky A, Alldred D. Medication review by pharmacists – the evidence still suggests benefit. *Pharm J* 2005; 274: 618–619.
43. Buisson, J. Vision for pharmacy – medication reviews in a GP surgery. *Pharm J* 2004; 272: 155.
44. Suchowersky O, deVries JD. Interaction of fluoxetine and selegiline. *Can J Psychiatry* 1990; 35: 571–572.

9

Further resources

This section lists a variety of sources of information and advice. Many of these are valuable to patients, their families and carers, as well as to healthcare professionals. The details for each of the sources listed were correct at the time of going to press, but obviously some changes may occur.

Organisations and websites

Parkinson's Disease Society
215 Vauxhall Bridge Road
London
SW1V 1EJ
UK
Tel: +44 (0)20 7931 8080; +44 (0)80 8000303 (helpline)
Fax: +44 (0)20 7233 9908
Email: enquiries@parkinsons.org.uk
Website: www.parkinsons.org.uk

The Parkinson's Disease Society is the leading charity in the UK committed to supporting people with Parkinson's disease, their families, friends and carers. Established in 1969 it now has 30 000 members, and over 300 branches and support groups throughout the country. The society provides information, advice and support not only to patients and their families, but also to health and social services professionals. Each year the society funds research into the causes of Parkinson's disease and potential cures, as well as helping to optimise use of treatments currently available.

Parkinson's Disease Society Scotland Office
Forsyth House
Lommond Court
Castle Business Park
Stirling
FK9 4TU
UK
Tel: +44 (0)1786 433811
Fax: +44 (0)1786 431811
Email: pds.scotland@parkinsons.org.uk
Website: www.parkinsons.org.uk

See details under Parkinson's Disease Society above for details of activities and services available.

Parkinson's Disease Society Wales Office
Maritime Offices
Woodland Terrace
Maesycoed
Pontypridd
CF37 1DZ
UK
Tel: +44 (0)1443 404916
Fax: +44(0)1443 408970
Email: pds.wales@parkinsons.org.uk
Website: www.parkinsons.org.uk

See details under Parkinson's Disease Society above for details of activities and services available.

Parkinson's Disease Society Northern Ireland Office
Dunsilly Lodge
Dunsilly
Antrim
BT41 2JH
UK
Tel: +44 (0)2894 428928
Fax: +44 (0)2894 428928
Email: rhamill@parkinsons.org.uk

Special Parkinson's Research Interest Group (SPRING)
PO Box 440
Horsham
W Sussex
RH13 0LA
UK
Tel: +44 (0)1403 730163
Email: secretary@spring.parkinsons.org.uk
Website: http://spring.parkinsons.org.uk

The Special Parkinson's Research Interest Group was set up by the Parkinson's Disease Society with the aim of accelerating research into Parkinson's disease. The group tries to improve co-ordination and increase funding for research into the disease and ultimately finding a cure.

Younger Parkinson's Network (YPN)
PO Box 33209
London
SW1V 1WH
UK
Tel: +44 (0)808 800 0303
Website: http://yap-web.net

The Younger Parkinson's Network has been established by the Parkinson's Disease Society. The website has particular focus on Parkinson's disease occurring in the younger age group and provides news items, details of events and has a FAQs section.

European Parkinson's Disease Association (EPDA)
4 Golding Road
Sevenoaks
Kent
TN13 3NJ
UK
Tel: +44 (0)1732 457683
Mobile: +44 (0)7787 554856
Fax: +44 (0)1732 457683
Email: lizzie@epda.eu.com
Website: www.epda.eu.com

The James Parkinson Centre
Camborne-Redruth Community Hospital
Redruth
Cornwall
TR15 3ER
UK
Website: www.pdcornwall.org.uk

The aims of this centre are to provide help to people in Cornwall who have Parkinson's disease or related disorders; to establish a community resource centre; and to advance the education of the public by increasing awareness of the disease and its implications.

British Geriatrics Society – Parkinson's Disease Section
Marjory Warren House
31 St John's Square
London
EC1M 4DN
UK
Tel: +44 (0)20 7608 1369
Fax: +44 (0)20 7608 1041
Email: info@pdsection.org.uk
Website: www.pdsection.org.uk

The Parkinson's disease section of the British Geriatrics Society site was established to help identify and co-ordinate interest and expertise in the field of Parkinson's disease amongst healthcare professionals. There is a particular focus on older people with the disease. A forum exists to promote discussion in service developments, audit and research.

World-wide Education and Awareness for Movement Disorders (WEMOVE)
204 W 84th Street
New York
NY 10024
USA
Tel: +1 800 437 6682; +1 212 875 8312
Email: wemove@wemove.org
Website: www.wemove.org

The website provides a comprehensive resource of information on a range of movement disorders including Parkinson's disease and symptoms associated with the disease, such as bradykinesia, tremor and restless legs syndrome.

American Parkinson Disease Association
135 Parkinson Avenue
Staten Island
NY 10305
USA
Tel: +1 718 981 8001; +1 800 223 2732
Fax: +1 718 981 4399
E-mail: apda@apdaparkinson.org
Website: www.apdaparkinson.org

The website provides general information for patients and healthcare professionals as well as news updates.

MouseCage Software House
(Software for people with hand tremor to help control their computer mouse)
67 Lansbury Avenue
Chadwell Heath
Romford, Essex
RM6 6SD
UK
Tel: +44 (0)7739 252 046
Fax: +44 (0)871 733 5278
Website: www.mousecage.org

MouseCage computer software is designed to help people who have hand tremor to control a computer mouse. It is suitable for people with essential tremor, Parkinson's disease, multiple sclerosis and other conditions resulting in tremor. A downloadable free trial version is available. It is available for computers running Microsoft Windows 2000 and Windows XP.

The Cure Parkinson's Trust (supported by Movers & Shakers)
Email: info@cureparkinsons.org.uk
Website: www.cureparkinsons.org.uk

The Cure Parkinson's Trust funds a number of research projects. The trust also hosts scientific forums, believing that communication within the scientific community is essential. By bringing researchers together for focused discussion on specific areas better progress can be made. The website provides details.

National Parkinson Foundation (NPF)
1501 NW Ninth Avenue
Bob Hope Road
Miami
FL 33136-1494
USA
Tel: +1 800 327 4545; +1 305 243 6666
Fax: +1 305 243 5595
Email: contact@parkinson.org
Website: www.parkinson.org

The National Parkinson Foundation (NPF) supports research related to Parkinson's disease, patient care, education and training. The foundation produces a number of leaflets. A large number of healthcare professions have taken part in their Allied Team Training for Parkinson (ATTP) Program. A biannual international symposium is held on research topics where researchers from around the world present and discuss the latest developments in the field of Parkinson's disease.

Parkinson's Disease Foundation
1359 Broadway
Suite 1509
New York
NY 10018
USA
Tel: +1 800 457 6676; +1 212 923 4700
Fax: +1 212 923 4778
Email: info@pdf.org
Website: www.pdf.org

The Parkinson's Disease Foundation (PDF) is involved in Parkinson's disease research, patient education and patient advocacy. Funding is provided for scientific research, and financial support given to patients, their families and carers. This extensive website provides new items and information on research which is under way. The Expert Resource Centre section of the site provides hundreds of frequently asked questions and answers about Parkinson's disease, which are listed by category.

The Parkinson Alliance
Post Office Box 308
Kingston
New Jersey
NJ 08540
USA
Tel: +1 800 579 8440; +1 609 688 0870
Fax: +1 609 688 0875
Email: admin@parkinsonalliance.net
Website: www.parkinsonalliance.net

The Parkinson Alliance is an organisation committed to raising funds to help finance research to find the cause and cure for Parkinson's disease. Copies of *The Catalyst* (their regular newletter) can be accessed via the website.

Young Onset Parkinson's Association (YOPA)
22136 Westheimer Parkway #343
Katy
Texas
77450 8296
USA
Tel: +1 888 937 9672
Email: directors@yopa.org
Website: www.yopa.org

The mission of the Young Onset Parkinson's Association (YOPA) is 'to serve all young-onset Parkinson's patients, particularly the recently diagnosed, by actively searching for them and providing them with empathy, information, an affiliation with others like themselves, a connection with the young-onset community, and a larger voice in advocacy'. The website provides a good up-to-date news section, message board and chat room, and links to other useful sites are listed.

Michael J Fox Foundation for Parkinson's Research
Grand Central Station
PO Box 4777
New York
NY 10163
USA
Tel: +1 800 708 7644; +1 212 509 0995
Website: www.michaeljfox.org

The Michael J Fox Foundation for Parkinson's Research is dedicated to the development of a cure for Parkinson's disease. It raises substantial funds to facilitate research in this endeavour. The website is very comprehensive and provides extensive up-to-date information on all aspects of Parkinson's disease, its treatment and research.

"James", a site about Parkinson's Disease
Website: http://james.parkinsons.org.uk/

This website provides details about Parkinson's disease, where patients can get support and information about coping with its effects. It is a project of the Adrienne Coles Memorial Trust (a trust dedicated to Parkinson's Disease information on the internet).

Appendix A

James Parkinson's description and treatment of the shaking palsy (Parkinson's disease)

An extract from Chapter I of *An Essay on the Shaking Palsy* by James Parkinson published in 1817: Definition – history – illustrative cases

So slight and nearly imperceptible are the first inroads of this malady, and so extremely slow is its progress, that it rarely happens, that the patient can form any recollection of the precise period of its commencement. The first symptoms perceived are, a slight sense of weakness, with a proneness to trembling in some particular part; sometimes in the head, but most commonly in one of the hands and arms. These symptoms gradually increase in the part first affected; and at an uncertain period, but seldom in less than twelve months or more, the morbid influence is felt in some other part. Thus assuming one of the hands and arms to be first attacked, the other, at this period becomes similarly affected. After a few more months the patient is found to be less strict than usual in preserving an upright posture: this being most observable whilst walking, but sometimes whilst sitting or standing. Sometime after the appearance of this symptom, and during its slow increase, one of the legs is discovered slightly to tremble, and is also found to suffer fatigue sooner than the leg of the other side: and in a few months this limb becomes agitated by similar tremblings, and suffers a similar loss of power.

Hitherto the patient will have experienced but little inconvenience and befriended by the strong influence of habitual endurance, would perhaps seldom think of this being the subject of disease, except when reminded of it by the unsteadiness of his hand, whilst writing or employing himself in any nicer kind of manipulation. But as the disease proceeds, similar employments are accomplished with considerable difficulty, the hand failing to answer with exactness to the dictates of the will. Walking becomes a task which cannot be performed without considerable attention. The legs are not raised to that height, or with that promptitude which the will directs, so that the utmost care is necessary to prevent frequent falls.

At this period the patient experiences much inconvenience, which unhappily is found daily to increase. The submission of the limbs to the directions of the will can hardly ever be obtained in the performance of the most ordinary offices of life. The fingers cannot be disposed of in the proposed directions, and applied with certainty to any proposed point. As time and the disease proceed, difficulties increase: writing can now be hardly at all accomplished; and reading, from the tremulous motion, is accomplished with some difficulty. Whilst at meals the fork not being duly directed frequently fails to raise the morsel from the plate: which, when seized, is with much difficulty conveyed to the mouth. At this period the patient seldom experiences a suspension of the agitation of his limbs. Commencing, for instance in one arm, the wearisome agitation is borne until beyond sufferance, when by suddenly changing the posture it is for a time stopped in that limb, to commence, generally, in less than a minute in one of the legs, or in the arm of the other side. Harassed by this tormenting round, the patient has recourse to walking, a mode of exercise to which the sufferers from this malady are in general partial; owing to their attention being thereby somewhat diverted from their unpleasant feelings, by the care and exertion required to ensure its safe performance.

But as the malady proceeds, even this temporary mitigation of suffering from the agitation of the limbs is denied. The propensity to lean forward becomes invincible, and the patient is thereby forced to step on the toes and fore part of the feet, whilst the upper part of the body is thrown so far forward as to render it difficult to avoid falling on the face. In some cases, when this state of the malady is attained, the patient can no longer exercise himself by walking in his usual manner, but is thrown on the toes and forepart of the feet; being, at the same time, irresistibly impelled to take much quicker and shorter steps, and thereby to adopt unwillingly a running pace. In some cases it is found necessary entirely to substitute running for walking; since otherwise the patient, on proceeding only a very few paces, would inevitably fall.

In this stage, the sleep becomes much disturbed. The tremulous motion of the limbs occur during sleep, and augment until they awaken the patient, and frequently with much agitation and alarm. The power of conveying the food to the mouth is at length so much impeded that he is obliged to consent to be fed by others. The bowels, which had been all along torpid, now, in most cases, demand stimulating medicines of very considerable power: the expulsion of the faeces from the rectum sometimes requiring mechanical aid. As the disease proceeds towards its last stage, the trunk is almost permanently bowed, the muscular power is more decidedly diminished, and the tremulous agitation becomes violent. The patient walks now with great difficulty, and unable any longer to support himself with his stick, he dares not venture on this exercise, unless assisted by an attendant, who walking backwards before him, prevents his falling forwards, by the pressure of his hands against the fore part of his shoulders. His words are now scarcely intelligible; and he is not only no longer able to feed himself, but when the food is conveyed to the mouth, so much are the actions of the muscles of the tongue, pharynx, &c. impeded by impaired action and perpetual agitation, that the food is with difficulty retained in the mouth until masticated; and then as difficultly swallowed. Now also, from the same cause, another very unpleasant circumstance occurs: the saliva fails of being directed to the back part of the fauces, and hence it is continually draining from the mouth, mixed with the particles of food, which he is no longer able to clear from the inside of the mouth.

An extract from Chapter V: Considerations respecting the means of cure

In such a case then, at whatever period of the disease it might be proposed to attempt the cure, blood should first be taken from the upper part of the neck, unless contra-i[n]dicated by any particul[ar] circumstance. After which vesicatories should be applied to the [sa]me part, and a purulent discharge obtained by appropriate use of the Sabine Liniment;[a] having recourse to the application of a fresh blister, when from the diminution of the discharging surface, pus is not secreted in a sufficient quantity. Should the blisters be found too inconvenient, or a sufficient quantity of discharge not be obtained thereby, an issue of at least an inch and a half in length might be established on each side of the vertebral columna, in its superior part. These, it is presumed, would be best formed with caustic and kept open with any proper substance*.

---

*   Cork, which has been hitherto neglected, appears to be very appropriate to this purpose. It possesses lightness, softness, elasticity and sufficient firmness; and is also capable of being readily fashioned to any convenient form. The form which it seems would be best adapted to the part, is that of an almond, or of the variety of bean called scarlet bean; but at least an inch and a half in length.

Note

a   A remedy prepared from the tops of the conifer, *Juniperus sabina*. The liniment was also used for treating syphilitic warts. Taken internally it caused irritation of the gastrointestinal tract, often so severe that death resulted.

Appendix B

Interactions involving drugs commonly used in the treatment of Parkinson's disease

This appendix provides basic guidance on the interactions that may occur between treatments for Parkinson's disease and other drugs. Although comprehensive, the listings do not provide details of all interactions that may potentially occur. Care should be taken to check under a category of drug (e.g. antimuscarinic, antipsychotic) as well as the name of a specific drug. The potential for an interaction does not necessarily mean that the combination must be avoided altogether in clinical practice. However, at the very least, extra care should be taken and the patient monitored for signs of an adverse interaction occurring.

Amantadine

Interacting drugs	Effects of interaction
Antimuscarinics: atropine, benzatropine, dicycloverine, flavoxate, glycopyrronium, hyoscine, ipratropium, orphenadrine, oxybutynin, procyclidine, propantheline, tiotropium, tolterodine, trihexphenidyl, trospium	Increased likelihood of antimuscarinic side-effects occurring
Antipsychotics: amisulpiride, aripiprazole, benperidol, chlorpromazine, clozapine, flupentixol, fluphenazine, haloperidol, levomepromazine, olanzapine, pericyazine, perphenazine, pimozide, pipotiazine, prochlorperazine, promazone, quetiapine, risperidone, sertindole, sulpiride, trifluoperazine, zotepine, zuclopenthixol	Increased likelihood of extrapyramidal side-effects occurring
Bupropion	Increased likelihood of adverse effects such as nausea, vomiting, and neuropsychiatric events
Domperidone	Increased likelihood of extrapyramidal side-effects occurring

Memantine	Increased likelihood of central nervous system (CNS) side-effects occurring; also may increase dopaminergic effects
Methyldopa	Increased likelihood of extrapyramidal side-effects; also methyldopa may decrease dopaminergic effects
Metoclopramide	Increased likelihood of extrapyramidal side-effects occurring
Tetrabenazine	Increased likelihood of extrapyramidal side-effects occurring

Apomorphine

Interacting drugs	Effects of interaction
Antipsychotics: amisulpiride, aripiprazole, benperidol, chlorpromazine, clozapine, flupentixol, fluphenazine, haloperidol, levomepromazine, olanzapine, pericyazine, perphenazine, pimozide, pipotiazine, prochlorperazine, promazone, quetiapine, risperidone, sertindole, sulpiride, trifluoperazine, zotepine, zuclopenthixol	Antipsychotic drugs may reduce the effectiveness of apomorphine
Entacapone	Possible increase in the effects of apomorphine
Memantine	May increase dopaminergic effects
Methyldopa	May decrease dopaminergic effects

Bromocriptine

Interacting drugs	Effects of interaction
Alcohol	Increased likelihood of side-effects occurring
Antipsychotics: amisulpiride, aripiprazole, benperidol, chlorpromazine, clozapine, flupentixol, fluphenazine, haloperidol, levomepromazine, olanzapine, pericyazine, perphenazine, pimozide, pipotiazine, prochlorperazine, promazone, quetiapine, risperidone, sertindole, sulpiride, trifluoperazine, zotepine, zuclopenthixol	Antipsychotic drugs may reduce the effectiveness of bromocriptine

Isometheptene	Increased likelihood of side-effects occurring
Macrolide and ketolide antibiotics: azithromycin, clarithromycin, erythromycin, telithromycin	Possible increase in side-effects of bromocriptine due to an increase in blood levels
Memantine	May increase dopaminergic effects
Methyldopa	May decrease dopaminergic effects
Octreotide	Possible increase in side-effects of bromocriptine due to an increase in blood levels
Phenylpropanolamine	Increased likelihood of side-effects occurring

Cabergoline

Interacting drugs	*Effects of interaction*
Antipsychotics: amisulpiride, aripiprazole, benperidol, chlorpromazine, clozapine, flupentixol, fluphenazine, haloperidol, levomepromazine, olanzapine, pericyazine, perphenazine, pimozide, pipotiazine, prochlorperazine, promazone, quetiapine, risperidone, sertindole, sulpiride, trifluoperazine, zotepine, zuclopenthixol	Antipsychotic drugs may reduce the effectiveness of bromocriptine
Macrolide and ketolide antibiotics: azithromycin, clarithromycin, erythromycin, telithromycin	Possible increase in side-effects of cabergoline due to an increase in blood levels
Memantine	May increase dopaminergic effects
Methyldopa	May decrease dopaminergic effects

Entacapone

Interacting drugs	*Effects of interaction*
Antidepressants	Little information available, but caution advised with monoamine oxidase inhibitors (MAOIs), tricyclics, selective serotonin reuptake inhibitors (SSRIs) and venlafaxine
Apomorphine	The effects of apomorphine may be increased due to entacapone interfering with its metabolism

Iron	The effectiveness of entacapone may be reduced due to orally administered iron preparations decreasing its absorption due to chelation. This effect can be avoided by taking the drugs 3 h apart
Memantine	May increase dopaminergic effects
Methyldopa	The effects of methyldopa may be increased due to entacapone interfering with its metabolism; also methyldopa may decrease dopaminergic effects
Rasagiline	The blood levels, and therefore the effectiveness, of rasagiline may be reduced by entacapone
Selegiline	To reduce the likelihood of troublesome side-effects, the dosage of selegiline should not exceed 10 mg daily
Sympathomimetics: adrenaline (epinephrine), dobutamine, dopamine, dopexamine, isoprenaline, noradrenaline (norepinephrine)	The effects of sympathomimetics may be increased due to entacapone interfering with their metabolism. Entacapone blocks the action of catechol-O-methyl transferase (COMT) and therefore may interfere with the metabolism of drugs containing a catechol group
Warfarin	The anticoagulant effects of warfarin may be increased by entacapone. The international normalised ratio (INR) should be monitored when commencing or stopping treatment or when dosage is changed

Levodopa

Interacting drugs	Effects of interaction
Angiotensin-converting enzyme (ACE) inhibitors: captopril, cilazapril, enalapril, fosinopril, imidopril, lisinopril, moexipril, perindopril, quinapril, ramipril, transolapril	Increased likelihood of hypotension
Alpha-blockers: doxazosin, indoramin, prazosin, terazosin	Increased likelihood of hypotension
Angiotensin II receptor antagonists: candesartan, eprosartan, irbesartan, losartan, olmesartan, telmisartan, valsartan	Increased likelihood of hypotension

Antimuscarinics: atropine, benzatropine, dicycloverine, flavoxate, glycopyrronium, hyoscine, ipratropium, orphenadrine, oxybutynin, procyclidine, propantheline, tiotropium, tolterodine, trihexphenidyl, trospium	Any drug with antimuscarinic properties may decrease the absorption of levodopa
Antipsychotics: amisulpiride, aripiprazole, benperidol, chlorpromazine, clozapine, flupentixol, fluphenazine, haloperidol, levomepromazine, olanzapine, pericyazine, perphenazine, pimozide, pipotiazine, prochlorperazine, promazone, quetiapine, risperidone, sertindole, sulpiride, trifluoperazine, zotepine, zuclopenthixol	Antipsychotics can potentially decrease the effects of levodopa
Baclofen	Increased likelihood of agitation, confusion and hallucinations
Benzodiazepines: alprazolam, chlordiazepoxide, clobazam, clonazepam, diazepam, flurazepam, loprazolam, lorazepam, lormetazepam, midazolam, nitrazepam, oxazepam, temazepam	Benzodiazepines can potentially decrease the effects of levodopa
Beta-blockers: acebutolol, atenolol, bisporolol, carvedilol, celiprolol, esmolol, labetolol, metoprolol, nadolol, nebivolol, oxprenolol, pindolol, propranolol, sotalol, timolol	Increased likelihood of hypotension
Bupropion	Increased likelihood of adverse effects such as nausea, vomiting and neuropsychiatric events
Calcium channel blockers: amlodipine, diltiazem, felodipine, isradipine, lacidipine, lercandipine, nicardipine, nifedipine, nimodipine, nisoldipine, verapamil	Increased likelihood of hypotension
Clonidine	Increased likelihood of hypotension
Diazoxide	Increased likelihood of hypotension
Diuretics	Increased likelihood of hypotension
General anaesthetics (volatile liquid): desflurane, halothane, isoflurane, sevoflurane	Risk of cardiac arrhythmias
Iron	Iron preparations may decrease the absorption of levodopa
Memantine	Memantine may increase the effects of levodopa
Methyldopa	Increased likelihood of hypotension; also methyldopa may decrease the effects of levodopa

MAOI antidepressants: isocarboxazid, moclobemide, phenelzine, tranylcypromine	Risk of hypertensive crisis (wait for at least two weeks after stopping an MAOI before commencing treatment with levodopa)
Moxonidine	Increased likelihood of hypotension
Nitrates: glyceryl trinitrate, isosorbide dinitrate, isosorbide mononitrate	Increased likelihood of hypotension
Phenytoin	Phenytoin may decrease the effects of levodopa
Selegiline	Selegiline enhances the effects of levodopa (the dosage of levodopa should be reduced as necessary)
Vasodilators: hydralazine, minoxidil, sodium nitroprusside	Increased likelihood of hypotension

NB: pyridoxine can reduce the effects of levodopa, but only when it is given without a peripheral dopa decarboxylase inhibitor. Since in clinical practice levodopa is always given with a peripheral dopa decarboxylase inhibitor (benserazide or carbidopa), this potential interaction is of academic interest only.

Lisuride

Interacting drugs	*Effects of interaction*
Antipsychotics: amisulpiride, aripiprazole, benperidol, chlorpromazine, clozapine, flupentixol, fluphenazine, haloperidol, levomepromazine, olanzapine, pericyazine, perphenazine, pimozide, pipotiazine, prochlorperazine, promazone, quetiapine, risperidone, sertindole, sulpiride, trifluoperazine, zotepine, zuclopenthixol	Antipsychotic drugs may reduce the effectiveness of lisuride
Memantine	May increase dopaminergic effects
Methyldopa	May decrease dopaminergic effects

Pergolide

Interacting drugs	*Effects of interaction*
Antipsychotics: amisulpiride, aripiprazole, benperidol, chlorpromazine, clozapine, flupentixol, fluphenazine,	Antipsychotic drugs may reduce the effectiveness of bromocriptine

haloperidol, levomepromazine,
olanzapine, pericyazine, perphenazine,
pimozide, pipotiazine, prochlorperazine,
promazone, quetiapine, risperidone,
sertindole, sulpiride, trifluoperazine,
zotepine, zuclopenthixol

Memantine	May increase dopaminergic effects
Methyldopa	May decrease dopaminergic effects
Metoclopramide	May decrease dopaminergic effects

Pramipexole

Interacting drugs	Effects of interaction
Antipsychotics: amisulpiride, aripiprazole, benperidol, chlorpromazine, clozapine, flupentixol, fluphenazine, haloperidol, levomepromazine, olanzapine, pericyazine, perphenazine, pimozide, pipotiazine, prochlorperazine, promazone, quetiapine, risperidone, sertindole, sulpiride, trifluoperazine, zotepine, zuclopenthixol	Antipsychotic drugs may reduce the effectiveness of bromocriptine
Cimetidine	Possible increase in side-effects of ropinirole due to an increase in blood levels caused by a reduction in excretion
Memantine	May increase dopaminergic effects
Methyldopa	May decrease dopaminergic effects

Rasagiline

Interacting drugs	Effects of interaction
Dextromethorphan	Increased risk of adverse effects
Entacapone	Entacapone my reduce blood levels of rasagiline and therefore its effectiveness
Fluoxetine	Risk of serotonin syndrome (CNS excitation, hypertension) (wait for at least 5 weeks after stopping fluoxetine before commencing treatment with rasagiline. Wait for at least 2 weeks after stopping rasagiline before commencing treatment with fluoxetine)

Fluvoxamine	Risk of serotonin syndrome (CNS excitation, hypertension) (wait for at least 1 week after stopping fluvoxamine before commencing treatment with rasagiline. Wait for at least 2 weeks after stopping rasagiline before commencing treatment with fluvoxamine)
Memantine	May increase dopaminergic effects
Methyldopa	Methyldopa may decrease dopaminergic effects
MAOI antidepressants: isocarboxazid, moclobemide, phenelzine, tranylcypromine	Risk hypertensive crisis (wait for at least 2 weeks after stopping rasagiline before commencing treatment with MAOIs)
Pethidine	CNS toxicity may occur; pethidine should not be given until after 2 weeks of stopping rasagiline
SSRI antidepressants: citalopram, escitalopram, fluoxetine, fluvoxamine, paroxetine, sertraline	Risk of serotonin syndrome (CNS excitation, hypertension) see also separate entries for fluoxetine and fluvoxamine
Sympathomimetics: adrenaline (epinephrine), dobutamine, dopamine, dopexamine, isoprenaline, noradrenaline (norepinephrine)	Increased risk of side-effects
Tramadol	Risk that CNS toxicity and hyperpyrexia may occur. Avoid combined use if possible, otherwise monitor patient for signs of an interaction occurring
Tricyclic antidepressants: amitriptyline, amoxapine, clomipramine, dosulepin, doxepin, imipramine, lofepramine, nortriptyline, trimipramine	Risk of CNS toxicity
Venlafaxine	Risk of serotonin syndrome (CNS excitation, hypertension) (wait for at least 1 week after stopping venlafaxine before commencing treatment with rasagiline. Wait for at least 2 weeks after stopping rasagiline before commencing treatment with venlafaxine)

Ropinirole

Interacting drugs	Effects of interaction
Antipsychotics: amisulpiride, aripiprazole, benperidol, chlorpromazine, clozapine, flupentixol, fluphenazine, haloperidol, levomepromazine, olanzapine, pericyazine, perphenazine, pimozide, pipotiazine, prochlorperazine, promazone, quetiapine, risperidone, sertindole, sulpiride, trifluoperazine, zotepine, zuclopenthixol	Antipsychotic drugs may reduce the effectiveness of ropinirole
Memantine	May increase dopaminergic effects
Methyldopa	May decrease dopaminergic effects
Metoclopramide	May decrease dopaminergic effects
Oestrogens	Increased risk of ropinirole toxicity due to increased blood levels

Rotigotine

Interacting drugs	Effects of interaction
Alcohol	Increased likelihood of side-effects occurring
Antipsychotics: amisulpiride, aripiprazole, benperidol, chlorpromazine, clozapine, flupentixol, fluphenazine, haloperidol, levomepromazine, olanzapine, pericyazine, perphenazine, pimozide, pipotiazine, prochlorperazine, promazone, quetiapine, risperidone, sertindole, sulpiride, trifluoperazine, zotepine, zuclopenthixol	Antipsychotic drugs may reduce the effectiveness of rotigotine
Memantine	May increase dopaminergic effects
Methyldopa	May decrease dopaminergic effects

Selegiline

Interacting drugs	Effects of interaction
Dopamine	Risk of hypertensive crisis
Entacapone	To reduce the likelihood of troublesome side-effects, the dosage of selegiline should not exceed 10 mg daily if given to patients receiving entacapone
Fluoxetine	Risk of serotonin syndrome (CNS excitation, hypertension) (wait for at least 5 weeks after stopping fluoxetine before commencing treatment with selegiline. Wait for at least 2 weeks after stopping selegiline before commencing treatment with fluoxetine)
Fluvoxamine	Risk of serotonin syndrome (CNS excitation, hypertension) (wait for at least 1 week after stopping fluvoxamine before commencing treatment with selegiline. Wait for at least 2 weeks after stopping selegiline before commencing treatment with fluvoxamine)
Memantine	May increase dopaminergic effects
Methyldopa	Methyldopa may decrease dopaminergic effects
Moclobemide	Increased risk of adverse effects
Oestrogens	Increased risk of selegiline toxicity due to increased blood levels
Paroxetine	Risk of serotonin syndrome (CNS excitation, hypertension) (wait for at least 2 weeks after stopping paroxetine before commencing treatment with selegiline. Wait for at least 2 weeks after stopping selegiline before commencing treatment with paroxetine)
Pethidine	CNS toxicity and hyperpyrexia may occur. Avoid combined use
Progestogens	Increased risk of selegiline toxicity due to increased blood levels
SSRI antidepressants: citalopram, escitalopram, fluoxetine, fluvoxamine, paroxetine, sertraline	Risk of serotonin syndrome (CNS excitation, hypertension) see also separate entries for fluoxetine, fluvoxamine, paroxetine, sertraline

Sertraline	Risk of serotonin syndrome (CNS excitation, hypertension) (wait for at least 2 weeks after stopping sertraline before commencing treatment with selegiline. Wait for at least 2 weeks after stopping selegiline before commencing treatment with sertraline)
Tramadol	Risk that CNS toxicity and hyperpyrexia may occur. Avoid combined use if possible, otherwise monitor patient for signs of an interaction occurring
Venlafaxine	Risk of serotonin syndrome (CNS excitation, hypertension) (wait for at least 1 week after stopping venlafaxine before commencing treatment with selegiline. Wait for at least 2 weeks after stopping selegiline before commencing treatment with venlafaxine)

Tolcapone

Interacting drugs	*Effects of interaction*
Antidepressants	Little information available, but caution advised with MAOIs, tricyclics, SSRIs and venlafaxine
Memantine	May increase dopaminergic effects
Methyldopa	Methyldopa may decrease dopaminergic effects
Warfarin	The anticoagulant effects of warfarin may be increased by tolcapone. The international normalised ratio (INR) should be monitored when commencing or stopping treatment or when dosage is changed

Appendix C

Adverse effects associated with drugs used to treat Parkinson's disease

Note: commonly occurring adverse reactions are often mild to moderate. Furthermore, many appear in the early stages of treatment and often reduce in severity or disappear as therapy continues.

Gastrointestinal

	Co-careldopa	Co-beneldopa	Bromocriptine	Cabergoline	Lisuride	Pergolide	Pramipexole	Ropinirole	Apomorphine	Rotigotine	Amantadine	Selegiline	Rasagiline	Entacapone	Tolcapone	Trihexyphenydil
Nausea	✓	✓	✓	✓	✓	✓	✓	✓	✓	✓	✓	✓	✓	✓	✓	✓
Vomiting	✓	✓	✓	✓	✓	✓		✓	✓	✓	✓		✓	✓	✓	✓
Constipation			✓	✓	✓	✓	✓			✓	✓	✓	✓	✓	✓	✓
Diarrhoea	✓	✓				✓				✓	✓	✓		✓	✓	
Anorexia	✓	✓								✓	✓	✓	✓	✓	✓	
Dry mouth			✓							✓	✓	✓	✓	✓	✓	✓
Dyspepsia				✓		✓				✓			✓		✓	
Duodenal ulcer	✓	✓														
Gastric ulcer			✓													
Gastrointestinal bleeding	✓	✓	✓													
Dark saliva	✓	✓														
Alterations in taste	✓	✓														

Nervous system

	Co-careldopa	Co-beneldopa	Bromocriptine	Cabergoline	Lisuride	Pergolide	Pramipexole	Ropinirole	Apomorphine	Rotigotine	Amantadine	Selegiline	Rasagiline	Entacarpone	Tolcapone	Trihexyphenydil
Dyskinesia	√	√	√	√	√	√	√	√	√	√		√	√	√	√	
Headache	√	√	√		√		√	√		√	√	√	√		√	
Somnolence	√	√	√	√	√	√	√	√	√	√				√	√	
Drowsiness	√	√	√	√	√	√	√	√	√	√						
Sudden onset of sleep	√		√		√	√	√	√	√	√				√	√	
Vertigo										√		√	√			
Light-headedness	√	√									√					
Ataxia											√					
Slurred speech										√	√					
Convulsions										√	√					
Paraesthesia	√															
Neuroleptic malignant syndrome	√a	√a	√a			√a								√a	√a	

a On reducing dose or stopping treatment.

Psychiatric

	Co-careldopa	Co-beneldopa	Bromocriptine	Cabergoline	Lisuride	Pergolide	Pramipexole	Ropinirole	Apomorphine	Rotigotine	Amantadine	Selegiline	Rasagiline	Entacapone	Tolcapone	Trihexyphenidyl
Confusion	✓	✓	✓	✓		✓	✓	✓	✓	✓	✓	✓		✓	✓	✓
Hallucinations	✓	✓	✓	✓	✓	✓	✓	✓	✓	✓	✓	✓	✓	✓	✓	✓
Insomnia	✓	✓				✓	✓			✓	✓	✓		✓	✓	✓
Sleep disorders										✓	✓	✓		✓	✓	
Dream abnormalities	✓	✓					✓			✓			✓		✓	
Restlessness										✓	✓					✓
Agitation	✓	✓									✓	✓				
Anxiety	✓	✓						✓		✓	✓	✓				✓
Euphoria	✓	✓								✓	✓					✓
Psychosis	✓	✓										✓				
Pathological gambling				✓			✓	✓								
Depression	✓	✓								✓	✓		✓			
Memory impairment										✓	✓					✓
Loss of concentration										✓	✓					
Lethargy					✓											

Cardiovascular

	Co-careldopa	Co-beneldopa	Bromocriptine	Cabergoline	Lisuride	Pergolide	Pramipexole	Ropinirole	Apomorphine	Rotigotine	Amantadine	Selegiline	Rasagiline	Entacarpone	Tolcapone	Trihexyphenydil
Orthostatic hypotension	✓	✓	✓	✓	✓	✓	✓	✓	✓	✓	✓	✓	✓	✓	✓	
Bradycardia								✓								
Cardiac irregularities	✓	✓		✓		✓						✓	✓			✓
Palpitations	✓	✓				✓				✓	✓	✓				✓
Hypertension	✓	✓								✓		✓				
Angina pectoris				✓								✓	✓			
Myocardial infarction						✓							✓			
Tachycardia	✓	✓								✓						
Cerebrovascular accident													✓			
Livedo reticularis											✓					
Pericardial fibrosis			✓	✓	✓	✓										
Pericarditis			✓	✓		✓										
Raynaud's syndrome			✓	✓	✓	✓										
Cardiac valvulopathy				✓		✓										

Respiratory

	Co-careldopa	Co-beneldopa	Bromocriptine	Cabergoline	Lisuride	Pergolide	Pramipexole	Ropinirole	Apomorphine	Rotigotine	Amantadine	Selegiline	Rasagiline	Entacapone	Tolcapone	Trihexyphenidyl
Dyspnoea						✓			✓	✓		✓				
Nasal congestion			✓													
Rhinitis						✓										
Cough										✓						
Hiccup										✓						
Pleural effusion			✓	✓	✓	✓										
Pleural fibrosis			✓	✓	✓	✓										
Pleuritis			✓	✓	✓	✓										
Pulmonary fibrosis			✓	✓	✓	✓										
Bronchospasm									✓a							

a Due to sodium metabisulphite included in the formulation of the injection.

Skin

	Co-careldopa	Co-beneldopa	Bromocriptine	Cabergoline	Lisuride	Pergolide	Pramipexole	Ropinirole	Apomorphine	Rotigotine	Amantadine	Selegiline	Rasagiline	Entacapone	Tolcapone	Trihexyphenidyl
Rash	✓	✓	✓		✓	✓				✓	✓	✓	✓	✓	✓	✓
Alopecia			✓									✓				
Flushing	✓	✓		✓												
Hyperhydrosis	✓	✓								✓		✓		✓	✓	
Dark sweat	✓															
Diaphoresis											✓					
Pruritis	✓	✓								✓						
Contact dermatitis										✓			✓			
Exanthema										✓	✓					
Photosensitisation											✓					
Erythema										✓						
Urticaria									✓							
Local reaction										✓				✓	✓	
Vesicle									✓	✓						
Induration and nodules									✓	✓						
Tenderness									✓							
Panniculitis	✓	✓														
Skin cancer													✓			

Haematological

	Co-careldopa	Co-beneldopa	Bromocriptine	Cabergoline	Lisuride	Pergolide	Pramipexole	Ropinirole	Apomorphine	Rotigotine	Amantadine	Selegiline	Rasagiline	Entacapone	Tolcapone	Trihexyphenidyl
Leucopenia	✓	✓									✓		✓			
Haemolytic anaemia	✓	✓							✓							
Non-haemolytic anaemia	✓	✓														
Thrombocytopenia	✓	✓										✓				
Agranulocytosis	✓	✓														
Leucocytopenia												✓				
Eosinophilia									✓							

Urogenital

	Co-careldopa	Co-beneldopa	Bromocriptine	Cabergoline	Lisuride	Pergolide	Pramipexole	Ropinirole	Apomorphine	Rotigotine	Amantadine	Selegiline	Rasagiline	Entacapone	Tolcapone	Trihexyphenydil
Urine discolouration	✓	✓												✓	✓	
Dark urine	✓	✓														
Urinary retention	✓										✓	✓				✓
Urinary incontinence	✓										✓					
Urinary urgency	✓															
Erectile dysfunction										✓						

Musculoskeletal

	Co-careldopa	Co-beneldopa	Bromocriptine	Cabergoline	Lisuride	Pergolide	Pramipexole	Ropinirole	Apomorphine	Rotigotine	Amantadine	Selegiline	Rasagiline	Entacapone	Tolcapone	Trihexyphenidyl
Leg cramps			✓													
Arthralgia										✓		✓	✓			
Arthritis													✓			
Tenosynovitis													✓			
Joint swelling										✓						

Pain

	Co-careldopa	Co-beneldopa	Bromocriptine	Cabergoline	Lisuride	Pergolide	Pramipexole	Ropinirole	Apomorphine	Rotigotine	Amantadine	Selegiline	Rasagiline	Entacapone	Tolcapone	Trihexyphenidyl
Neck pain													✓			
Back pain												✓				
Chest pain												✓	✓		✓	
Abdominal pain			✓	✓	✓	✓		✓		✓			✓	✓	✓	

Eye/vision

	Co-careldopa	Co-beneldopa	Bromocriptine	Cabergoline	Lisuride	Pergolide	Pramipexole	Ropinirole	Apomorphine	Rotigotine	Amantadine	Selegiline	Rasagiline	Entacapone	Tolcapone	Trihexyphenidyl
Blurred vision										✓	✓					✓
Diplopia						✓										
Visual disorder							✓			✓	✓					
Reduced visual acuity																
Oculogyric crises	✓										✓					
Corneal lesions											✓					
Corneal epithelial oedema																
Conjunctivitis													✓			
Photopsia										✓						

Other adverse reactions

	Co-careldopa	Co-beneldopa	Bromocriptine	Cabergoline	Lisuride	Pergolide	Pramipexole	Ropinirole	Apomorphine	Rotigotine	Amantadine	Selegiline	Rasagiline	Entacapone	Tolcapone	Trihexyphenidyl
Fatigue			√				√	√		√	√	√		√	√	
Oedema				√			√	√		√	√	√				
Dizziness	√		√	√	√	√	√	√		√	√	√		√	√	√
Syncope	√	√		√		√		√		√		√				
Allergic reaction									√a	√						
Weight loss										√			√	√	√	
Malaise					√								√			
Flu syndrome						√							√		√	
Fever										√			√			
Increased libido	√	√					√	√								
Decreased libido							√	√								
Hepatitis														√	√	
Rhabdomyolysis														√	√	
Retroperitoneal fibrosis			√	√	√	√										

a Due to sodium metabisulphite included in the formulation of the injection.

Abnormal laboratory results

	Co-careldopa	Co-beneldopa	Bromocriptine	Cabergoline	Lisuride	Pergolide	Pramipexole	Ropinirole	Apomorphine	Rotigotine	Amantadine	Selegiline	Rasagiline	Entacarpone	Tolcapone	Trihexyphenidyl
Raised liver enzymes	✓	✓				✓					✓	✓	✓	✓	✓	
Raised serum uric acid	✓	✓														
Raised blood urea nitrogen	✓	✓														

Appendix D

Parkinson's disease and driving

There are a number of issues that a person with Parkinson's disease needs to consider if intending to drive. Many of the drugs used can adversely affect the patient's ability to drive or carry out other tasks that require mental alertness. Not only do some drugs cause confusion and drowsiness, which means that driving and similar activities must be avoided, but sudden onset of sleep without warning has been associated with a number of drugs used in the treatment of Parkinson's disease. However, medication is not the only issue; the symptoms of the disease itself can clearly have important implications for driving as outlined below.

Driver and Vehicle Licensing Authority

As is the case with a number of neurological conditions, a patient is required to inform the Driver and Vehicle Licensing Authority (DVLA) if they have been diagnosed with Parkinson's disease. The DVLA will normally send to the patient a form known as 'PK1', which has to be completed and returned. Amongst other details that have to be provided, the patient has to indicate which of the following symptoms they experience:

- involuntary movements
- slowness of reaction times
- pain and/or muscle cramps in the limbs
- difficulty in concentration
- problems with memory
- episodes of confusion
- excessive daytime sleepiness.

It is advisable for patients who do suffer with any of these symptoms to provide further details explaining why they believe their fitness to drive is not compromised despite indicating that one or more of the symptoms is a feature of their condition. Details of treatments, including dosages, also have to be given, together with consent for further medical information and opinion to be provided by the patient's doctors or specialists.

Many patients are permitted to drive despite their diagnosis of Parkinson's disease, but clearly this depends on the nature and severity of symptoms they suffer. Normally a license is granted for 3 years, at which time the situation is reviewed. Where there is uncertainty about a patient's ability to drive safely, a special driving assessment may be carried out at a specialist driving centre or mobility assessment centre. Normally there would be a charge for this. Sometimes a patient may want to be assessed if the DVLA decides not to allow them to continue driving and they wish to appeal against the decision. In England and Wales the DVLA must be notified of the intention to appeal within 6 months of the decision. In Scotland, notification must be made within 21 days.

Insurance

A patient with Parkinson's disease must inform their insurance company that they have this condition, and at least third-party insurance cover must be held, otherwise it would be illegal to drive on public roads even if a licence is processed. An insurance policy would normally be invalidated if the driver failed to notify the company of any disabilities or serious illness. An insurance company will often continue to provide cover, but sometimes they will increase the cost of the premiums that must be paid. The rates charged by insurance companies can vary considerably, so a patient may be well advised to seek several quotations.

Special help

Some patients who are permitted to continue driving are eligible for certain types of assistance – either financial or practical. Their vehicle may be exempted from road tax and a blue badge may be granted which greatly assists by allowing a vehicle to be parked free of charge and, in some circumstances, in places where parking is not normally permitted. It should be noted that the person does not themself need to be a driver in order to be issued with a blue badge; the badge can be used in any car in which they are travelling. The Motability scheme provides exemption of value added tax (VAT) on adaptation work that needs to be carried out on a vehicle and subsequent maintenance and repairs.

Glossary

Action tremor: a tremor which occurs in a limb during an action, such as reaching out with the arm to touch an object; it may also affect the voice.

Akathisia: a feeling of restlessness and being unable to sit still.

Anosmia: reduced sense of smell.

Anticholinergic: A drug which blocks impulses in cholinergic nerves (those in which acetylcholine is the neurotransmitter).

Aphonia: inability of phonation; the patient knows what they wish to say and is able to articulate, but their voice is inaudible (loss of voice).

Athetoid: slow involuntary writhing, twisting movements, especially severe in the hands.

Basal ganglia: a group of nuclei in the brain including the caudate, putamen, globus pallidus, substantia nigra and subthalamic nucleus. The basal ganglia interconnect with the cerebral cortex, thalamus and brainstem, and are associated with the control of motor function, cognition, emotions and learning.

Bradykinesia: abnormal slowness of movement.

Caeruloplasmin: a globulin in plasma, involved with the transport of copper in the body; levels are reduced in Wilson's disease.

Catecholamines: a group of compounds, including adrenaline (epinephrine), noradrenaline (norepinephrine) and dopamine, the molecular structures of which include a catechol portion.

Catechol-O-methyl transferase (COMT): an enzyme involved in the breakdown of catecholamines such as adrenaline (epinephrine), noradrenaline (norepinephrine) and dopamine.

Choreiform: continuous involuntary rapid jerky movements affecting the limbs and the face.

Cogwheel rigidity: an erratic, jerky movement (e.g. of the arm) due to tremor superimposed on rigidity, seen when the muscle is passively stretched.

COMT inhibitors: drugs such as entacapone and tolcapone that inhibit the enzyme catechol-O-methyl transferase.

Contralateral: on the opposite side of the body.

Corpus striatum: part of the basal ganglia comprising the globus pallidus and striatum.

CT scan: computerised tomography – a method of imaging in which the absorption of X-ray beams projected through a body plane are computed to produce a cross-sectional picture of the part of the body being scanned (also known as CAT scan – computerised axial tomography).

Dat scan: A type of SPECT imaging using a ^{123}I-derivative to label presynaptic dopamine reuptake sites. Used to assess the integrity of the dopaminergic nigrostiatal system (see also single photon emission computed tomography (SPECT)).

Deep brain stimulation (DBS): application of electrical impulses to specific parts of the brain via implanted electrodes. Used for treating Parkinson's disease and essential tremor.

Dopa: dihydroxyphenylalanine – the amino acid precursor of dopamine (the neurotransmitter depleted in certain parts of the brain in Parkinson's disease). The drug levodopa (L-dopa) is converted to dopamine in the body.

Dopa decarboxylase: the enzyme which catalyses the conversion of dopa to the neurotransmitter dopamine.

Dopamine: a neurotransmitter which in Parkinson's disease is depleted in certain parts of the brain.

Dopaminergic: a neural pathway in which dopamine is the neuro-transmitter; or a drug which stimulates dopamine receptors or increases the amount of dopamine released at synapses.

Dysarthria: slurred speech caused by difficulty in controlling the muscles used when speaking, which results in problems articulating words.

Dyskinesia: distorted or impaired voluntary movement.

Dysphagia: difficulty in swallowing.

Dysphasia: impaired production of language and/or impaired understanding of language due to loss of co-ordination and failure to arrange words in the correct order.

Dysphonia: reduced volume of the voice due to the inability to phonate sufficiently, often resulting in hoarseness.

Dystonia: contraction of muscles in part of the body, resulting in a persistent posture or movement.

Extrapyramidal motor system: areas of the brain (basal ganglia, thalamus, brainstem nuclei) involved in the control of posture and movement.

Festinating gait: a term used to describe a type of walking where the patient involuntarily shuffles with increasing speed in an attempt to keep up with the forward momentum of the body; typically seen in patients with Parkinson's disease.

FP-CIT SPECT: a particular type of SPECT imaging using labelled cocaine derivatives such as ^{123}I-FP-CIT (see also Dat scan).

Glial cell line-derived neurotrophic factor (GDNF): a protein which enhances the survival of certain neurons such as the dopaminergic neurons affected by Parkinson's disease.

Globus pallidus: part of the basal ganglia.

Glutamatergic: a neural pathway in which glutamate is the neurotransmitter; or a drug which stimulates glutamate receptors or increases the amount of glutamate released at synapses.

Hypokinesia: reduction in movement.

Hyposmia: reduced sense of smell.

Ipsilateral: on the same side of the body.

Lead-pipe rigidity a rigidity which feels smooth, unlike the jerky rigidity resulting from superimposed tremor (cogwheel rigidity).

Lewy bodies: round microscopic protein structures found in certain nerve cells affected by Parkinson's disease; named after a German pathologist.

Magnetic resonance imaging (MRI) scan: a method of imaging in which an external magnetic field is directed to part of the body enabling visualisation of soft tissue due to variations in the resonance of hydrogen atoms in different environments.

Micrographia: handwriting which has become smaller than normal, or which decreases in size from normal to minute as it is written.

Monoamine oxidase inhibitor (MAOI): a drug which inhibits the enzyme monoamine oxidase thereby increasing the levels of catecholamines in the central nervous system.

MPTP: 1-methyl-4-phenyl-1,2,3,6-tetrahydropyridine, a compound which is metabolised by monoamine oxidase into MPP^+; it produces a parkinsonian syndrome similar to Parkinson's disease.

Myoclonus: muscle contractions which are shock-like and erratic in rhythm and amplitude.

Nigrostriatal pathway: the dopaminergic neural pathway connecting the substantia nigra with the striatum; in Parkinson's disease, dopamine deficiency occurs in this pathway.

NMDA receptors: N-methyl-D-aspartate receptors are found in certain pathways in the brain, and activated by the amino acid neurotransmitter glutamate.

Nocturia: frequent urination at night.

Pallidal stimulation: a type of deep brain stimulation where electrical impulses are applied to the pallidus via implanted electrodes.

Pallidotomy: a surgical lesioning procedure used to ablate part of the pallidus thereby reducing its activity.

Paraesthesia: altered sensation such as tingling, prickling or burning.

Paralysis agitans: the term used in the 19th century for what is now known as Parkinson's disease.

Parkinsonism: conditions which produce symptoms that are associated with Parkinson's disease, including hypokinesia, tremor and rigidity.

Peripheral dopa decarboxylase inhibitor: a drug which blocks the actions of the enzyme dopa decarboxylase in the body apart from the brain (e.g. carbidopa, benserazide).

Pharmacist with special interest (PhwSI):   the framework for establishing pharmacists with special interests was launched by the Department of Health in 2006.

Pharmacogenetic: a term used to describe differing responses to drugs in individuals due to genetic variation.

Positron emission tomography (PET) scan: a method of imaging which measures the concentration of a pre-administered positron-emitting radioisotope that selectively concentrates in certain tissues of the body (see Plate 4).

Postural tremor: a tremor that occurs when a particular position is maintained by the patient, for example in an outstretched arm.

Resting tremor: a tremor that occurs when part of the body is at rest, for example in a relaxed and supported arm. In Parkinson's disease this tremor is usually between 4 and 5 Hz.

Serotonergic: a neural pathway in which serotonin is the neurotransmitter; or a drug which stimulates serotonin receptors or increases the amount of serotonin released at synapses.

Shaking palsy: the term used in James Parkinson's original publication *Essay on the Shaking Palsy* in which he describes the condition now known as Parkinson's disease.

Sialorrhoea: producing excessive amounts of saliva.

Single photon emission computed tomography (SPECT):   a method of imaging in which a gamma camera detects a pre-administered gamma photon-emitting radio nucleotide, generating a set of two-dimensional images that are computed to produce a three-dimensional view.

Substantia nigra: the deepest structure of the basal ganglia from which the dopaminergic pathway affected by Parkinson's disease passes to the striatum.

Subthalamic nucleus: an oval-shaped area of grey matter in the caudal part of the subthalamus (the ventral part of the thalamus).

Subthalamic stimulation: a type of deep brain stimulation where electrical impulses are applied to the subthalamic nucleus via implanted electrodes.

Subthalamotomy: a surgical lesioning procedure used to ablate part of the subthalamic nucleus thereby reducing its activity.

Thalamic stimulation: a type of deep brain stimulation where electrical impulses are applied to the thalamus via implanted electrodes.

Thalamotomy: a surgical lesioning procedure used to ablate part of the thalamus thereby reducing its activity; it is effective for reducing tremor.

Transcranial electric polarisation (TCEP):   a non-invasive procedure where a weak electrical current (e.g. 2 mA) is passed via electrodes on the scalp; it has been researched as a possible treatment for Parkinson's disease.

Transcranial magnetic stimulation (TMS):   stimulating neurons in the brain by non-invasively applying electric currents induced by electromagnetic induction. Repetitive transcranial magnetic stimulation (rTMS) has been used in the treatment of a number of conditions including Parkinson's disease.

Tremor: an involuntary trembling or quivering.

Index

Plate references are in **bold**, figures and tables are in *italics*